CANCER ETIOLOGY, DIAGNOSIS AND TREATMENTS

ORAL SQUAMOUS CELL CARCINOMA

FROM DIAGNOSIS TO TREATMENT

Cancer Etiology, Diagnosis and Treatments

Additional books and e-books in this series can be found on Nova's website under the Series tab.

CANCER ETIOLOGY, DIAGNOSIS AND TREATMENTS

ORAL SQUAMOUS CELL CARCINOMA

FROM DIAGNOSIS TO TREATMENT

MATTHEW RABIN
EDITOR

nova
Medicine & Health
New York

Library of Congress Cataloging-in-Publication Data

ISBN: 978-1-53619-895-9

Published by Nova Science Publishers, Inc. † New York

CONTENTS

PREFACE

This book consists of five chapters that describe the diagnosis and treatment of oral squamous cell carcinoma (OSCC), which is the most common malignant epithelial neoplasm affecting the oral cavity. Chapter one deals with different potentially malignant disorders in the development of OSCC, diagnostic methods of OSCC, the pertinence of biomarkers in OSCC therapy, classification of biomarkers, existing biomarkers in different stages of OSCC and the challenges of developing new biomarkers. Chapter two is focused on principles, systems, technologies, therapeutic approaches, safety and toxicity and patents comprising drug delivery systems for local oral squamous cell carcinoma treatment. Chapter three aims to highlight a detailed critical review of previous literature on putative cancer stem cell pathways for oral carcinoma and draw interest in targeting the most common cancer stem cell markers as a therapeutic regimen for oral cancer preneoplastic tumors, metastasis, and treatment progression. Chapter four aims to cover the recent developments in nanotechnology-based drug delivery systems, advanced nanomedicines and their diagnostics as well as therapeutic applications in OSCC. Finally, chapter five aims to elaborate on the importance of biomarkers as an early diagnostic tool in detecting oral squamous cell carcinoma.

Chapter 1 - Oral Cancer is the sixth most common type of cancer worldwide and 90% of it is represented by Oral Squamous Cell Carcinoma

(OSCC). India has the highest prevalence of OSCC as per the World Oral Health Report. OSCC has few risk factors associated with it such as high metastasis rate, high probability of recurrence, less survival rate and lack of public awareness. Despite many advancements in therapeutic strategies, there is a tremendous increase in the mortality and morbidity rate due to the availability of tobacco and related products that elevate the occurrence of the disease. The majority of patients are diagnosed and treated for this disease at the terminal stages (III or IV). These are the main reasons for the escalating mortality rates. Due to this, there is an immense necessity for early diagnosis of OSCC which should be given utmost importance. Biomarkers are indispensable biological molecules that can be used to identify normal cellular alterations. Histological examination using biomarkers is considered as one of the most reliable technique for the diagnosis of OSCC. These biomarkers can also be analyzed by other means such as solid biopsy and liquid biopsy which contains DNA, RNA or proteins used for examining the expression pattern of particular genes or proteins. There are three broad categories of biomarker discoveries: Genomic, Proteomic and Metabolomic which is expressed during progression and metastasis of OSCC. This chapter deals with different potentially malignant disorders in the development of OSCC, diagnostic methods of OSCC, the pertinence of biomarker in OSCC therapy, classification of biomarkers, existing biomarkers in different stages of OSCC and the challenges of developing new biomarkers.

Chapter 2 - Oral squamous cell carcinoma is the third most common type of malignancy in developing countries and the eighth most common in developed countries. The rate survival is poor when there is late detection of these lesions. The development of oral mucosal drug delivery systems may be quite useful as treatment and as adjuvant of oral cancer. This chapter is focused on principles, systems, technology, therapeutic approaches, safety and toxicity and patents comprising drug delivery systems for local oral squamous cell carcinoma treatment. In this context, the most valuable and up-to-date oral drug delivery systems for oral squamous cell carcinoma were discussed. Some aspects and definitions were revised in terms of oral mucosal environment, challenges, and benefits of local treatment of oral squamous cell carcinoma, as well as the characteristics of the active pharmaceutical ingredients. The strategies to foster the drug delivery, the advances in both *in vitro* and *in vivo* activity, and patents and registered products in the market aiming local treatment of oral squamous cell carcinoma were considered.

Chapter 3 - Recurrence of tumors despite chemotherapy represents a profound medical condition with cancer of the oral cavity. Cancer stem cells (CSCs) have been recognized to orchestrate metastasis and facilitate tumor development in oral squamous cell carcinoma *via* the capability of self-renewal and proliferation to generate downstream progenitor cells and cancer cells. This chapter aims to highlight a detailed critical review of previous literature on putative cancer stem cell pathways for oral carcinoma and draw interest in targeting the most common cancer stem cell markers as a therapeutic regimen for oral cancer preneoplastic tumors, metastasis, and treatment progression. Thus, targeting cancer stem cells may help overcome the tumor spread and therapeutic resistance by reversing the epithelial and EMT (epithelial-to-mesenchymal transition) subpopulations shifts.

Chapter 4 - Oral squamous cell carcinoma (OSCC) is the most common cancer worldwide. Several factors influence OSCC, tobacco use having a high impact on OSCC development. The prevention of OSCC may be possible by reducing exposure to the risk factors of OSCC. OSCC is the sixth most deadly cancer globally, owing to the drawback of the traditional approach in OSCC treatment and failure of diagnosis at an early stage. The primary stage of detection and a sedentary lifestyle mainly contributes to the morbidity and mortality of OSCC patients. In this scenario, nanotechnology gives a new direction for the treatment and diagnosis of oral cancer. Nanomedicine shows a highly promising result with low toxicity. The toxicity of nanomaterial can be controlled by improving functionalization and systematically minimizing toxicity. As a result, nanomaterial and nanomedicine becomes more biologically compatible. Nanomedicine-based targeted drug delivery to the tumor site releases therapeutic agents most effectively, possibly increasing the efficacy of nanomedicine. This book chapter aims to cover the recent developments in Nanotechnology-based drug delivery systems, advance nanomedicines (Nano-capsules, Gold nanoparticles, Quantum dots, and Carbon nanotubes) and their diagnostics as well as therapeutic applications in OSCC.

Chapter 5 - According to global cancer statistics 2018 (GLOBOCAN 2018), cancer is the second leading cause of death globally. Estimated 18.1 million new cancer cases and 9.6 million cancer deaths. It is most common in India, accounting for 120000 with 90% of oral squamous cell carcinoma (OSCC). The incidence and mortality rate of cancer has shown a sharp increase over the last two decades. Most oral cancers are not diagnosed at an early stage even though they are easily accessible under direct visual examination. Mortality rates remain unchanged despite vast advances in the field of oncology. Therefore, more intense efforts are required to fight against life-threatening diseases and to reduce morbidity and mortality rates. Biomarkers are powerful diagnostic tools that can be measured in bodily fluids such as blood, serum, plasma, and body secretions such as saliva. They release certain biochemical substances that are expressed in large quantities at the cell surface by malignant cells. The anatomical proximity of salivary biomarkers to oral cancer makes it the most accurate and specific diagnostic tool and it is a non-invasive alternative to serum testing. More than 100 salivary biomarkers have already been identified, including cytokines (IL-8, IL-1β, and TNF-a), P53, transferrin, DUSP, MMP, and LDH. In recent years due to the revolution in molecular biology, the development of valid biomarkers has been a breakthrough in the field of cancer research and care. Substantial progress has been made in the development and clinical application of biomarkers and matched targeted therapies. The recent emergence of highly selective technologies has provided global information to observe genetic and proteomic alterations and to facilitate the discovery of new biomarkers with improved sensitivity and specificity. The use of biomarker-based diagnostics for cancer includes non-invasive screening for early-stage disease, detection and localization, risk assessment, disease stratification and prognosis, response to therapy and, for those in remission, screening for disease recurrence. The current chapter aims to elaborate on the importance of biomarkers as an early diagnostic tool in detecting oral squamous cell carcinoma.

In: Oral Squamous Cell Carcinoma ISBN: 978-1-53619-895-9
Editor: Matthew Rabin

Chapter 1

Biomarkers in the Progression and Metastasis of Oral Squamous Cell Carcinoma

Bhuvanadas Sreeshma[1], Diveyaa Sivakumar[2], Dibyo Maiti[3] and Arikketh Devi*

Department of Genetic Engineering, Cancer Biology and Stem Cell Biology Lab, School of Bioengineering, College of Engineering and Technology, SRM Institute of Science and Technology, Kattankulathur, TamilNadu, India

Abstract

Oral Cancer is the sixth most common type of cancer worldwide and 90% of it is represented by Oral Squamous Cell Carcinoma (OSCC). India has the highest prevalence of OSCC as per the World Oral Health Report. OSCC has few risk factors associated with it such as high metastasis rate, high probability of recurrence, less survival rate and lack of public awareness. Despite many advancements in therapeutic strategies, there is a

---

* Corresponding Author's E-mail: devia@srmist.edu.in.

tremendous increase in the mortality and morbidity rate due to the availability of tobacco and related products that elevate the occurrence of the disease. The majority of patients are diagnosed and treated for this disease at the terminal stages (III or IV). These are the main reasons for the escalating mortality rates. Due to this, there is an immense necessity for early diagnosis of OSCC which should be given utmost importance. Biomarkers are indispensable biological molecules that can be used to identify normal cellular alterations. Histological examination using biomarkers is considered as one of the most reliable technique for the diagnosis of OSCC. These biomarkers can also be analyzed by other means such as solid biopsy and liquid biopsy which contains DNA, RNA or proteins used for examining the expression pattern of particular genes or proteins. There are three broad categories of biomarker discoveries: Genomic, Proteomic and Metabolomic which is expressed during progression and metastasis of OSCC. This chapter deals with different potentially malignant disorders in the development of OSCC, diagnostic methods of OSCC, the pertinence of biomarker in OSCC therapy, classification of biomarkers, existing biomarkers in different stages of OSCC and the challenges of developing new biomarkers.

Keywords: oral squamous cell carcinoma, OSCC, potentially malignant disorders, OSCC diagnostic methods, types of biomarker, biomarker classification

INTRODUCTION

Cancer is one of the most dreaded disease initiated by aberrant proliferation of cells possessing the ability to invade neighbouring organs and metastasizing to various parts of the body through different ways. Every year, more than million patients are affected by cancer worldwide. Among the various types of cancer, the incidence and mortality rates of Oral Squamous Cell Carcinoma (OSCC) is higher in the Asian continent, especially being one of the top three common cancer prevalent in South-Central Asia. In middle and low-income countries, specifically in India, men are more prone to this cancer due to the ease of availability and consumption of areca nut, smokeless tobacco and other related products (Petersen et al. 2009). OSCC includes cancer of the lips, tongue, cheeks, floor of the mouth, hard and soft palate, sinuses, pharynx or any other part of the oral cavity. According to the World Health Organization statistics, one-third of the OSCC cases are from India (World Health Organization 2016). It is estimated that this proportion may get doubled by 2030 (Varshitha et al. 2015). OSCC has multifactorial aetiology, where the challenges such as high recurrence rate, late diagnosis, patient negligence and 5-year survival rate contributes to the worsening of the disease and this has remained unchanged for the past few decades. The progression and metastasis of OSCC are primarily due to genetic as well as epigenetic changes combined with the environmental risk factors such as tobacco use, smoking, alcohol consumption, Human Papilloma Virus infection and chronic inflammation (B. Wang et al. 2013).

In OSCC, 90% of the deaths are due to metastasis especially when the patients do not respond to any of the treatment options. Though an examination of the oral cavity is quite easy by visualization, most of the OSCC cases are not identified at the early stages as it is mostly asymptomatic during this stage. (Hadzic et al. 2017). Even though numerous prognostic and diagnostic methods for several cancers have been identified so far, the early detection of OSCC remains cumbersome. Furthermore, Epstein et al., 2015 has reported that abundant cases show delayed or misdiagnosis of OSCC by dental and medical health care providers while some others alleged that there are some health complications due to osteonecrosis of the jaw (Epstein et al. 2015).

DEVELOPMENT OF ORAL SQUAMOUS CELL CARCINOMA

OSCC tumorigenesis reveals a sequence of histopathological events ranging from hyperplasia to dysplasia of differing aggressiveness to carcinoma in situ which subsequently progresses to invasive squamous cell carcinoma (Hunter, Parkinson, and Harrison 2005). According to Braakhuis et al., 2003, OSCC is initiated by a genetic alteration in a stem cell located in the basal cell layer of oral mucosa which turns out into a patch termed as a clonal unit containing stem cell with its daughter cells having the same genetic alteration. Later, this patch expands along with additional genetic variations in the region and these mucosal fields dominate the growth of normal epithelium and expand in its size. These regions are invisible in the beginning but may appear as oral patches later. Eventually, clonal selection results in the formation of carcinoma (Braakhuis, B. J., Tabor, M. P., Kummer, J. A., Leemans, C. R., & Brakenhoff, n.d.).

There are many Potentially Malignant Disorders (PMDs) that have a predisposition to reorganize into OSCC and these are the following:

1. Leukoplakia is common in men (54.2%) with around 80% of the cases leading to hyperkeratosis or acanthosis (Waldron and Shafer 1975). Bewley et al., 2017 has reported that this can lead to the formation of OSCC (Bewley and Farwell 2017), (Farooq and Bugshan 2020).
2. Proliferative Verrucous Leukoplakia (PVL) is a vigorous form of oral leukoplakia that forms white lesions which spreads slowly with a high rate of reappearance and malignancy (Thompson 2006). In addition, another study conducted by Bagán et al., 2004 showed similar results of a high probability of patients with PVL developing OSCC (Bagán et al. 2004).
3. Erythroleukoplakia is a condition of mixed red and white lesions appearing in the oral cavity. Abundant dysplastic lesions are seen in this condition when compared to leukoplakia (Bánóczy 1997).
4. Erythroplakia, a red coloured lesion, is considered a clinical finding of OSCC. Leukoplakia and erythroplakia are termed as predecessors of OSCC (Grajewski and Groneberg 2009). A study conducted by Yang et al., 2015 revealed that 91% of the samples are diagnosed as OSCC (51%), with 40% carcinoma in situ or severe dysplasia and 9% mild or moderate dysplasia (S. W. Yang et al. 2015).
5. Oral Lichen Planus (OLP) may persist for multiple years with periodic outbursts and remission. Although biopsies and histopathological examinations are recommended to diagnose this condition, there are no specific criteria to assess the risks associated with OLP. (Fitzpatrick, Hirsch, and Gordon 2014).

6. Oral Lichenoid Lesions (OLL) or Oral Lichenoid Reactions (OLR) are intra-oral red and white lesions with similar clinical features as OLP. These are induced by drugs or can develop in persons who are continuous betel-quid chewers. Later, OLL can transform into malignant OSCC (van der Meij, Mast, and van der Waal 2007).
7. Graft versus Host Disease (GvHD) is a condition caused as a result of allogeneic hematopoietic stem cell or bone marrow transplants. It is accompanied by numerous signs and symptoms and involves multifarious organ sites, frequently affecting the oral cavity (Schubert and Correa 2008). It has been reported that GvHD has the potential to invade and form aggressive OSCC (Mawardi et al. 2011).
8. Discoid Lupus Erythematosus (DLE) is a chronic autoimmune disorder with 20% of the patients manifesting oral lesions affecting buccal mucosa, palate and lips (Saman Warnakulasuriya 2018). The lower lip is the most commonly affected area in DLE mediated malignant transformation (Millard and Barker 1978).
9. Oral Submucous Fibrosis (OSF) is a chronic disease involving the lamina propria of oral mucosa. As the disease progresses, it affects deeper tissues in the oral submucosa resulting in loss of fibroelasticity (Saman Warnakulasuriya 2018). The severity of the disease includes difficulty in opening the mouth and the presence of numerous lesions of erythroplakia and leukoplakia (S. Warnakulasuriya 1987), (Kerr et al. 2011).
10. Epidermolysis Bullosa (EB) is a skin disease characterised by blisters and erosions in the oral mucosa. Even though EB is considered a potentially malignant disease, specific oral malignant lesions are not well characterized and the frequency of malignant transformation is comparatively less (Fine et al. 2009).
11. Leukokeratosis Nicotina Palatinae (LNP)/Palatal changes in reverse smokers is also another PMD that may transform to OSCC. Reverse smoking, is an unusual type of smoking in which the burned end of a rolled tobacco leaf termed as “chutta” (an Indian product) or cigarettes will be placed inside the mouth instead of the unsmoked

end. This type of habit is pervasive in many parts of India, Philippines, Panama, Colombia, Jamaica, Venezuela, Sardinia, Caribbean islands etc., Earlier research conducted by Gupta et al., in 1980 observed the presence of profuse PMDs in the oral palate in the course of a 10-year follow up (Gupta, Mehta, and Daftary 1980). This includes leukoplakia, mucosal nodularity, ulceration, yellowish-brown staining, erythema etc., which could develop into a malignancy.

12. Dyskeratosis congenital, a rare inherited condition of bone marrow failure shows oral leukoplakia as the most common symptom. These patients are more prone to develop malignancy (Bongiorno et al. 2017).
13. Actinic Cheilitis, achronic inflammation in lips, is caused due to prolonged exposure to solar ultraviolet radiation. Those who have less melanin content show significantly increased risk of developing this condition (Wood NH, Khammissa R, Meyerov R, Lemmer J, n.d.). During the disease progression, the ulcerative lesions may slowly develop, progress with inflammation, atrophy and finally, the loss of epithelium leads to the formation of OSCC (de Oliveira Ribeiro, da Silva, and Martins-Filho 2014).
14. Other PMDs include:
    a) Chronic Hyperplastic Candidiasis (CHC), also known by the term candidal leukoplakia is an oral candidiasis variant caused by *Candida albicans.* This condition is characterised by white patches in the oral mucosal layer. If the lesions are untreated, they may develop into OSCC (Shah et al. 2017).
    b) Syphilis is one of the main cause of cheilitis glandularis, which is a condition of hyperplasia of minor salivary glands that may progress to OSCC (Mortazavi, Baharvand, and Mehdipour 2014).
    c) Actinic Keratosis is an other intraepidermal skin tumour that can develop into SCC (Fuchs and Marmur 2007).
    d) Sideropenic Dysphagia, also known as Plummer-Vinson syndrome is a rare PMD characterized by dysphagia,

oesophageal webs and chronic iron deficiency anaemia. There are reports that this condition may also lead to the development of OSCC (Jessner et al. 2003).

LATEST DIAGNOSTIC METHODS

Despite the ease of clinical examination of the oral cavity, the majority of the PMDs are not diagnosed at their early stages and this is one of the reasons for the low survival rate of OSCC patients. In addition, lack of public awareness is also a crucial factor in OSCC diagnosis. Creating public awareness against the usage of tobacco-related products and reiterating the need for early diagnosis of OSCC by monitoring PMDs may effectively mitigate oral health problems (Macpherson et al. 2018), (Seki et al. 2011). Besides tumour size that plays a significant role in the prediction of OSCC, lymph node metastasis also is a decisive factor (S. F. Huang et al. 2012). Clinicians use the Tumor, Nodes and Metastasis (TNM) staging system to predict the tumour grade to date, but the unfortunate reality is that patients with identical TNM stages may exhibit different distinct clinical behaviours, treatment responses and patient outcomes (T. Y. Fu et al. 2016), (Oliveira-Costa et al. 2015), (Jerjes et al. 2010). Thus, multitude of varying clinico pathological parameters can be observed for OSCC with regard to its incidence, recurrence, disease progression, survival and metastasis. Some of these are:

1) Primary site of occurrence
2) Tumour size and volume (Depth of invasion)
3) Lymph Node Involvement
4) Metastasis (Distant/cervical)
5) Degree of differentiation
6) Invasive Front (Pattern of invasion)
7) Perineural/Endoneural Invasion
8) Gender
9) Age at the first occurrence

10) Race
11) Presence of dysplasia at the margin and severe dysplasia (SD)
12) Lymphovascular and nervous invasion
13) Bone/cartilage invasion
14) Tumour clearance

Although there are advancements in existing clinical treatments, the overall survival rates of OSCC patients remains unsatisfactory. Preliminary diagnosis of OSCC is one of the pre-eminent way to alleviate the high mortality and morbidity of OSCC. Some of the non-invasive techniques used for diagnosis and confirmation of OSCC are:

Vital Staining

These include some of the staining procedures followed using a collection of pigments that act on highly proliferative cells and neoplastic cells. A study highlighted the effective use of 5% acetic acid for OSCC diagnosis (Bhalang et al. 2008). Another research conducted by Sankaranarayanan et al., 2003 on cervical cancer stated that using 4% acetic acid is an effective diagnostic method with a sensitivity and specificity of 88% and 78% in particular (Sankaranarayanan et al. 2003).

Toluidine blue staining is another easy, affordable and sensitive staining technique for identifying early stages of OSCC and severe dysplasia (Mashberg 1981). This acidophilic metachromatic nuclear stain helps to differentiate the carcinoma in situ regions or invasive carcinoma regions from normal tissue by staining only the nucleus which has a rapid proliferation rate. This stain is highly specific and sensitive to malignant regions. 1% of Toluidine Blue solution added for 30 seconds gives 93.5% to 97.8% sensitivity of OSCC screening and specificity ranging from 73.3% to 92.9% (Rosenberg and Cretin 1989).

Methylene blue, an acidophilic dye penetrates into the cells containing a high amount of nucleic acid and shows variation in the uptake of stain between the normal and cancer cells (Y. W. Chen et al. 2007). Lugol's

Iodine staining has more affinity towards glycogen in epithelial cells and therefore it stains normal cells more when compared to the cancer cells which have less glycogen content. As per a study conducted by Epstein et al.,1992, it was stated that Lugol's Iodine can be used as a diagnostic procedure for oral malignancy (Epstein, Scully, and Spinelli 1992). The double staining procedure with Lugol's Iodine and Methylene Blue greatly improves the detection efficiency of OSCC (G. Peng et al. 2011). Du et al., 2007 proposed a promising staining technique with Rose Bengal stain for evaluation of OSCC (Du et al. 2007).

Oral Brush Biopsy

This simple, painless test is shown to have high sensitivity and specificity than surgical biopsies, ranging over 90%. Oral brush collects majority of the cells from the oral epithelium (Sciubba 1999), (Scheifele et al. 2004).

Saliva Based OSCC Diagnosis

This technique is an alternative for serum testing. Also, this is an effective diagnostic method for poor OSCC prognosis and to detect post-therapy status. Increased concentration of Cyfra 21-1, tissue polypeptide specific antigen (TPS), cancer antigen 125 (CA125) are a few of the antigens used for analysis (Handschel et al. 2007), (Zimmermann BG, n.d.). Liquid biopsy is one of the latest technology that makes use of saliva and is the most easily accessible, painless, low cost and helpful source of diagnostic and prognostic biomarker detection since it contains DNA, RNA, circulating tissue-derived cells, circulating tumour DNA, extracellular vesicles and miRNA.

Light-Based Detection System

Devices specially designed with light source work on the tissue reflectance and tissue auto-fluorescence principle to enhance oral cavity scrutiny. Autofluorescence technique is introduced in some devices to analyse oral cavity such as VELscope®, Identafi 3000® with high specificity (Hanken et al. 2013), (Rana et al. 2012). Narrowband imaging is a novel endoscopic visualization technique using light generated with optical interference filters with varied lower frequency spectral range. Bhatia et al., 2013 revealed that the use of narrowband imaging technology is one of the processes with high specificity, sensitivity, Positive Predictive Value (PPV), Negative Predictive Value (NPV) for diagnosing OSCC (Bhatia et al. 2013).

Other Light-Based Detection Systems include

- Ratio imaging
- Raman spectroscopy
- Elastic scattering spectroscopy
- Differential Path-Length Spectroscopy (DPS)
- Spectral Scatter Scanning System
- Nuclear Magnetic Resonance Spectroscopy (NMR)
- Optical Coherence Tomography
- Infrared Spectroscopy
- Confocal Endomicroscopy

Chemiluminescence Based Detection

ViziLite Plus® is a tissue reflectance-based device that uses a disposable chemiluminescent light packet. Microlux/DL® and Orascoptic DK® are devices that use a reusable LED (Light Emitting Diode) powered by a battery which provides light equivalent to blue-white light illumination (M.

W. Lingen et al. 2008), (Rethman et al. 2010). The sensitivity and specificity of chemiluminescent based detection cannot be accounted as these were only conducted on patients with visible lesions.

Histological and Cytological Techniques

Incisional (IB) or Excisional Biopsy (EB) is the best available diagnostic technique for OSCC. Histopathology can determine the severity of epithelial dysplasia, the foremost prognostic malignancy indicator. Furthermore, histopathology helps to identify OSCC even though no lesions are visible. A study conducted by Goodson et al., 2011 reported that histological examinations are more accurate, as even the severity of dysplasia can be distinguished properly. According to pathologists complete excision of OSCC lesion is indispensable to diagnose and to expedite early potential therapy of undetectable OSCC with severe dysplastic and neoplastic lesions (Goodson and Thomson 2011).

Cytopathology is the analysis of cell samples from oral mucosal surface collected by smears, scrapings, lavage etc., performed externally and using fine needle aspiration internally. Oral exfoliative cytology makes use of the cells that flake off from oral mucosa naturally or artificially and liquid-based cytology uses liquid medium for sampling, thence fixed to reduce sample degradation (M. W. Lingen et al. 2008). OralCDx® Brush Test system, Cytobrush®Plus GT are the types of specialized brushes which collect transepithelial cellular samples that contain cell clusters and free cells. There are innumerable literatures focussing on the efficacy and specificity of these systems (Fontes et al. 2013), (Delavarian et al. 2010).

Molecular Analysis

Oral Squamous Cell Carcinoma (OSCC) is a slowly progressing aggressive cancer with multifarious levels of expression of signature molecular markers throughout the stages. These signature molecular markers termed "biomarkers," are identified and their expression patterns are ascertained in every stage of OSCC to distinguish the tumour grading. Therefore, the necessity for identifying a reliable biomarker for OSCC to differentiate various stages of OSCC is inevitable. There are numerous categories of biomarkers that have been identified so far in OSCC.

EMINENCE OF BIOMARKERS IN OSCC THERAPY

OSCC grading using molecular methods is one of the promising tools which minimizes the discrepancy in histology (Bremmer et al. 2005). The escalation of genetic variations in pivotal genes designated as proto-oncogenes, which can transform into oncogenes, tumour suppressor genes and DNA repair genes altogether facilitates the malformation of cells by modulation of normal cell genotype and phenotype. In addition to this, a series of molecular events which accelerate the development of deformed, rapidly proliferating cells (M. Lingen et al. 2011) also occurs continuously and these genetic alterations form the basis of oral tumorigenesis. The precise knowledge of these changes on genetic, molecular or metabolic molecules and the cellular processes underlying carcinogenesis can pave the way towards understanding and earliest identification of OSCC.

The biomolecules generated by either tumour cells or other immune cells in the body in response to tumour development are called Cancer Biomarkers. It could be genes, gene products, cells, molecules, enzymes, hormones etc., that can be identified through tissues, blood, urine or other body fluids. These biomarkers are unique signature molecules that vary according to the type of cell it is derived from and may be released during OSCC initiation, development, progression and metastasis. Comprehending the oral tumorigenesis mechanism could explain the production and release of these markers into the blood or other body fluids in elevated amounts and its differential expression as cancer metastasizes. In addition to checking their presence or absence, the expression levels, activities of genes, proteins, molecular attributes etc., are also validated. Analysis of these candidate markers would facilitate and aid in understanding the molecular hallmarks of oral tumorigenesis. These molecular markers would also assist to anticipate, investigate and provide better knowledge on OSCC progression and metastasis. Moreover, the chromosomal aberrations corresponding to OSCC pathogenesis also needs to be analyzed and therefore it becomes a necessity to examine the predictive genetic markers for early detection, prognosis and predicting response to OSCC (M. Lingen et al. 2011). Biomarker analysis in OSCC plays a significant role in

- Evaluating the risk of developing cancer (Easton et al. 1995)
- Screening (K. Lin et al. 2008)
- Differential diagnosis (Lauritano et al. 2016), (Blatt et al. 2017)
- Determining the prognosis of the disease (Harishankar et al. 2019), (Z. Yang et al. 2019)
- Predicting therapy response (Rettori et al. 2013)
- Monitoring disease recurrence (Rettori et al. 2013), (Cristaldi et al. 2019)
- Monitoring the progression or regression of metastasis (Sowmya, Rao, and Prasad 2020)

An ideal biomarker should be precise enough to differentiate benign case from the malignant cancer and aggressive metastasized tumour. Also, it should be

- Organ or tissue–specific
- Proportional to tumour volume
- Exhibit short half-life
- Easily identifyable even if present at low levels in the serum of healthy individuals (exist quantitatively)
- Distinguish metastasis
- Standardized
- Reproducible
- Validated
- Cost-effective

- Obtain the sample for testing in a non-invasive manner
- Reliable
- Accurate
- Specific and sensitive (Henry and Hayes 2012), (Kamel HF, n.d.).

IDENTIFICATION OF CANDIDATE BIOMARKERS IN OSCC

Biomarkers are identified by copious molecular techniques such as Real-Time Polymerase Chain Reaction (RT-PCR), High throughput Next-Generation sequencing, DNA arrays, Gene Expression Arrays, Restriction Fragment Length Polymorphism (RFLP), Ribonucleoprotein Immunoprecipitation-gene chip, Cross-linking Immunoprecipitation, Liquid Chromatography, Nuclear Magnetic Resonance, Mass Spectroscopy, enzyme assays, Immunohistochemistry (IHC), multiplex IHC, Flow cytometry, mass cytometry, Fluorescent In-Situ Hybridization etc., The principle approach to identify a candidate biomarker is based on the understanding of tumour biology and the tumour microenvironment or the metabolism of the pharmaceutical agent. With the advent of novel technologies, the research on the identification of suitable biomarker for specific cancers is going on at a fast pace. However, there are several processes involved in identifying a potential biomarker before it is clinically applicable. Initially, a set of samples are analysed to test the potential of the novel biomarker. To validate the hypothesis, a sequence of experiments substantiating the importance of the biomarker needs to be performed. This will assist to establish the clinical use of these biomarkers and further investigations on analytical validity, clinical validity and clinical utility (Teutsch et al. 2010) should be assessed to finally authenticate its use as a biomarker.

Analytical validity is the verification of both the pre-analytical and analytical issues of the assay to approve the novel biomarker. This involves exploring the technical aspects of the biomarker assay that should meet certain criteria. Furthermore, it is critical to analyse sensitivity, specificity, the robustness of assay, accuracy and reproducibility in laboratories (Moore et al. 2013). If a technically valid assay has been developed, then it should undergo clinical validity testing to assess if it has any clinical or biological validity before recommending the biomarker directly for clinical care (Ransohoff and Gourlay 2010). Clinical utility is the final step before introducing the biomarker to patient care. This assessment includes confirming the effectiveness of biomarker and the benefit to harm ratio etc., (Allegra et al. 2009). The final process will be the clinical implementation with regulatory committee approval, commercialization, health insurance coverage and incorporation to practice guidelines (Goossens et al. 2015). Some of the different types of biomarkers available are:

Prognostic Biomarkers

It is based on the clinical or biological attributes, which provides information on the probability of OSCC outcomes such as disease progression, metastasis, recurrence, duration of life without regard to the treatment taken. Biomarkers generally have a degree of prognostic value equivalent to their predictive role and therefore there are chances that one gets dominated by the other. The prognostic biomarker which gets wrongly labelled as predictive may have deteriorative effects and may end up misinterpreting the benefits of the treatment. Correspondingly, the price of the drug will shoot up as the demand increases although it is not ideal for all patients (Ruberg and Shen 2015). The prognostic biomarkers in OSCC include Matrix Metallo Protease2 (MMP2), Matrix Metallo Protease1 (MMP1), Cadherin-1, mucin-1, p53, Epidermal Growth Factor Receptor (EGFR) etc., (Trivedi et al. 2011; G. Z. Huang et al. 2019; Wei et al. 2020; Jiang et al. 2015; Rivera et al. 2017).

Predictive Biomarkers

The predictive biomarker is a boon to the patient which aids in controlling the disease before it progresses. Assessing the risk of developing malignancy in a person can be determined by identifying the risk reduction strategies (lifestyle, prophylactic surgery, chemoprevention etc.,) or by more effective screening. This method is highly beneficial to patients who belong to the high-risk category than to the whole population. Thus, prognostic biomarkers help in determining the risk of developing OSCC by analysing the lifestyle, HPV status, genetic and epigenetic alterations.

Ballman et al., 2015 revealed that there exists certain ambiguity on the distinction between predictive biomarkers and prognostic biomarkers (Ballman 2015). The utilisation of biomarkers in OSCC treatment imparts a prognostic signal that could have an impact on personal, financial and ethical issues. The predictive biomarkers discovery has led to the observation that there is a lack of attention in *in-silico* studies (X. Su et al. 2008). The articles on subgroup discovery comprehend predictive biomarkers as an intermediate step in cancer prediction along with Interaction Trees (X. Su et al. 2008), SIDES (Lipkovich et al. 2011) and Virtual Twins (Foster, Taylor, and Ruberg 2011). A novel bioinformatics tool termed INFO+ developed by Konstantinos Sechidis et al., 2018 which can distinguish between the prognostic and predictive role of the biomarkers is advantageous in this regard (Sechidis et al. 2018).

Diagnostic Biomarkers

The biomarkers which are used for screening OSCC by distinguishing the various possibilities for differential diagnosis sometimes are referred to as detective biomarkers. For example, if a patient has oral lesions, then the patient will be advised to provide biopsy specimens for histological evaluation that can determine whether the tissue is cancerous, has infection, inflammation or any other benign process. Further, immunohistochemistry is performed also to identify the tissue of origin once the cancerous condition is confirmed (Lauritano et al. 2016), (Henry and Hayes 2012).

In addition, there are several studies to identify diagnostic biomarkers through different types of approaches including proteomics studies (Z. Yang et al. 2019), (R. Wang et al. 2018; Chu et al. 2019; Tung et al. 2013; Lai et al. 2010).

Pharmacodynamic Biomarkers

The biomolecules which indicate the effect of the drug on a target organism by evaluating the link between drug regimens, target effects and tumour responses are referred to as pharmacodynamics biomarkers. These help in drug development by measuring the molecular target status, pharmacokinetic parameters of drug exposure, pharmacodynamics endpoint of drug effects on targeted cells, pathway implications, assessment of downstream targets in the pathway, affected biological processes etc., and coupling novel drugs, combining targeted agents and optimizing schedules for combinational drug therapeutics. These biomarkers specifically play a crucial role in delivering targeted treatments by validating clinical pharmacodynamics biomarker assays in drug development. Major two programs where such biomarkers are intertwined include cancer imaging program and clinical assay laboratory which produce a robust and accurate measurement of drug effects in each patient thus supporting in NEXT drug development projects (Sarker and Workman 2006; Jackson 2012; Gainor, Longo, and Chabner 2014; "No Title," n.d.).

Risk Assessment Biomarkers

With the increase in the cost of healthcare and new targeted therapies, the use of biomarkers has emanated as a method for assessing the risk of OSCC occurrence and recurrence. There are few bioinformatics tools available to predict cancer risk management and using molecular biomarkers with these tools enables to optimize the available resources to control cancer progression by assessing the risk associated with the particular tumour stage and predicting the disease development (X. Li et al. 2011), (Preston 2006).

CLASSIFICATION OF OSCC BIOMARKERS

The broad classification of biomarkers according to the OSCC stages, type of biomolecules and its applications as listed in Table 1.

Table 1. Broad classification of biomarkers based on the Oral Squamous Cell Carcinoma stages, type of biomolecules and its applications

OSCC Biomarkers			
Based on the OSCC stages	**Based on biomolecules**		**Based on its applications**
Risk Assessment	Genomics 1. DNA Based	Loss of Heterozygosity/ Copy number variation	Imaging Biomarkers
Screening		Sequence variation	Pathological Biomarkers
Prediction		Epigenetic variation	*In-silico* Biomarkers
Patient Grouping		Genomic rearrangements	
Monitoring Therapy	2. DNA Type Based	Circulating Tumour DNA	
Staging		Circulating cell-free DNA	
Diagnosis		Mitochondrial DNA	
Prognosis	RNA Based	Circular RNA	
		Messenger RNA	
		Micro RNA	
		Long non-coding RNA	
	Proteomics	Proteins or enzymes	
		Peptides	
	Metabolomics	Metabolites	
		Carbohydrates	
		Lipids	

BIOMARKERS IN GENOMICS

There are some factors such as replication errors, ineffective DNA repair systems or cell cycle checkpoints, chromosomal instabilities and chromosomal aberrations, which are the possible genetic alterations that could lead to cell damage and result in oncogenesis (Lengauer, Kinzler, and Vogelstein 1998), (Janssen and Medema 2013). Microsatellites are highly polymorphic, short tandem repeat sequence of 2-6 base pairs in length existing throughout the genome. Microsatellite Instability (MSI) is a type of gene mutation where replication errors and dysfunction of mismatch repair leads to DNA sequence alterations (Yamamoto and Imai 2015). A study reported of higher incidence of MSI at D2S123 loci in patients with OSCC and they suggested that MSI could act as a diagnostic indicator (Panda et al. 2015). Some other studies also reported a similar conclusion that patients with MSI have a higher probability of OSCC recurrence (J. C. Lin et al. 2016). Loss of Heterozygosity (LOH) is a mechanism of tumour-suppressor gene inactivation by which the loss of a wild type allele of a chromosome changes a heterozygous somatic cell into a hemizygous cell (Happle 1999). It has been reported that the frequency of LOH is much more than MSI of upto 80% especially on chromosome arms 3p, 4q, 7q, 8q, 9p, 11q, 13q and 17p. These regions display abundance of tumour suppressor regions such as Transforming Growth Factor Beta Receptor 2 (TGFBR2) and Contactin 4 (CNTN4) on Chr. 3p and Lysine Demethylase 4C (KDM4C), Interleukin33 (IL33), Protein Tyrosine Phosphatase Receptor Type D (PTPRD), SH3 Domain Containing GRB2 Like 2, Endophilin A1 (SH3GL2), FRAS1 Related Extracellular Matrix 1 (FREM1) on Chr. 9p, or neighbouring Tumour suppressor genes (TSG) regions such as the cyclin-dependent kinase inhibitor 2A (p16/CDKN2) gene cluster, Tumor Suppressor Candidate 1 (TUSC1) and Doublesex And Mab-3 Related Transcription Factor 2 (DMRT2) (Chen et al. 2015). Some literature states that LOH can be considered as a biomarker for identifying invasive OSCC (Rao et al. 2018; Numasawa et al. 2005; Kayahara et al. 2001). Another interesting feature of OSCC is that the oral and maxillofacial regions in the human body is rich in blood supply and because of the physical stimulation of external immense pressure created, the oral cancer regions will deliver genetic material into blood circulation in the form of either tumour cells or microvesicles. The circulating tumour DNA (ctDNA) has the similar genetic feature as that of the tumour. Thus, the presence of ctDNA is used to diagnose the tumour which reduces the need of tissue biopsy. Its presence in the saliva is considered as one of the non-invasive liquid biopsy done on cancer samples (Bettegowda C, Sausen M, Leary RJ, Kinde I, Wang Y, Agrawal N, Bartlett BR, Wang H, Luber B, Alani RM, n.d.), (Babji et al. 2019).

Saliva contains copious components such as cellular debris, microorganisms, inorganic and organic molecules (Chiappin et al. 2007). Biomarkers are detectable more in saliva than in serum or plasma (Yuxuan Wang et al. 2015). Saliva also contains tumour-derived DNA secreted by exosomes or microvesicles (Principe et al. 2013).

Single Nucleotide Polymorphisms

Single nucleotide polymorphisms (SNPs) are defined as variations in a genetic sequence that affects only a single base in that sequence and is present in >1% of the population. SNPs are present throughout the entire human genome and is responsible for almost 90% of genetic variations that occurs in humans. Even though the majority of SNPs do not have any effect on normal cellular functions, some SNPs are involved in the development of various diseases including cancer. Such SNPs are usually present in genes that are involved in cell cycle regulation, cell metabolism, signalling pathways and DNA repair, thus interfering with normal cell function (Gayther et al. 2007; Grochola et al. 2010; J. Liu et al. 2014). Several studies have confirmed that certain SNPs have been associated with a higher risk of cancers including OSCC.

Table 2. The types of single nucleotide polymorphisms used as a biomarkers in Oral Squamous Cell Carcinoma

Genes	Population	SNPs	References
ATM Serine/Threonine Kinase (ATM)	Taiwan	rs189037 (G→A)	(Cao and Li 2006)
Cyclin D1-1	India	rs647451 (C→T)	(Murali et al. 2014)
Cyclin D2	India	rs3217901 (A→G)	(Murali et al. 2014)
Cyclin E	India	rs1406 (A→C)	(Murali et al. 2014)
Cyclin H	India	rs3093816 (A→G)	(Murali et al. 2014)
Cyclin-dependent kinase inhibitor (p27)	India	rs34329 (C→G)	(Murali et al. 2014)
Retinoblastoma *gene* (Rb1-1)	India	rs3092904 (T→A)	(Murali et al. 2014)
Transforming growth factor beta-1 (TGF-β1)	Taiwan	rs1800471 (G→C)	(Hsu et al. 2015)
Interleukin-4 *(IL-4)*	India	rs2070874 (T→C)	(Gaur et al. 2011)
Interleukin-6 *(IL-6)*	India	rs1800795 (G→C)	(Gaur et al. 2011)
Interleukin-10 *(IL-10)*	China	rs1800870 (A→G)	(J. G. Yao et al. 2008)
Interleukin-10	China	rs1800871 (A→C)	(J. G. Yao et al. 2008), (Niu et al. 2015), (Umare et al. 2020)
	China	rs1800872 (T→C)	
	China	rs1800896 (G→A)	
Interleukin-17A *(IL-17A)*	China	rs2275913 (A→G)	(N. Li et al. 2015)
Interleukin-17*F (IL-17F)*	China	rs2392084 (T→G)	(N. Li et al. 2015)
Interleukin-23R *(IL-23R)*	Taiwan	rs10889677 (C→A)	(Chien et al. 2012)
Survivin	Taiwan	rs9904341 (C→G)	(C. J. Weng et al. 2012)
Survivin	Taiwan	rs2071214 (A→G)	(C. J. Weng et al. 2012)
Survivin	Taiwan	rs10422489 (C→T)	(C. J. Weng et al. 2012)
Protein kinase 1 (AKT1)	Chinese	rs1130214 (G→T)	(Yun Wang et al. 2015)
	Chinese	rs3803300 (A→G)	
Human MutL homolog 1 (hMLH1)	India	rs1800734 (A→G)	(Jha et al. 2013)
Tumor Necrosis Factor Receptor Associated Factor (TRAF6)	China	rs5030486 (G→A)	(Yun Wang et al. 2014)
Vascular Endothelial Growth Factor (VEGF)	India	rs833061(C→T)	(Borase et al. 2015)
X-Ray repair cross-complementing protein 1 (XRCC1)	Thailand	rs1799782(G→A)	(Kietthubthew et al. 2006)
X-Ray repair cross-complementing protein 3 (XRCC3)	Thailand, Germany	rs861539(C→T)	(Kietthubthew et al. 2006), (Werbrouck et al. 2008)

Table 2. (Continued)

Genes	Population	SNPs	References
Xeroderma pigmentosum group D (XPD)	Chinese	- c.466 (C→A)	(Kietthubthew et al. 2006)
Caspase-7 (CASP7)	Indian, Portuguese	rs2227310(C→G)	(Datta et al. 2015), (Azevedo et al. 2019)
Caspase-10 (CASP10)	Indian	rs13010627 (G→A)	(Datta et al. 2015)
BH3 Interacting-domain death agonist (BID)	Indian	rs8190315(T→C)	(Datta et al. 2015)
Bcl-2-like protein 2 (BCL2L2)	Indian	rs1950252(A→G)	(Datta et al. 2015)

Specifically in OSCC, the associated SNPs have been detected in cell cycle and proliferation genes (Cao and Li 2006; Murali et al. 2014; Hsu et al. 2015), immune function-related genes (Gaur et al. 2011; J. G. Yao et al. 2008; N. Li et al. 2015; Chien et al. 2012), apoptosis genes (C. J. Weng et al. 2012; Yun Wang et al. 2015) and DNA repair genes (Jha et al. 2013). Identifying such SNPs will be useful in the development of biomarkers with diagnostic or prognostic values. Some of them are listed in Table 2.

Chromosomal Rearrangements

Chromosomal rearrangements have been well described in OSCC (Papanikolaou et al. 2018; Németh et al. 2019; Martin et al. 2008). Such chromosomal aberrations have been studied using low-resolution methods including Fluorescence in Situ Hybridization (FISH), spectral karyotyping and cytogenetic techniques. Now, using next-generation sequencing (NGS), the detection of chromosomal rearrangements can be performed in a faster and more efficient way. Chromosomal rearrangements that are specific to tumour tissues have the potential to be used as biomarkers for cancer detection. Such biomarkers would be useful for monitoring cancer progression, understanding tumour response to cancer therapies, detecting cancer recurrences and for long term patient management as well.

One type of chromosomal rearrangements includes recurrent gene fusions that are repeatedly observed in a specific type of tumour. Initially, recurrent gene fusions were only observed in hematologic malignancies, but recently recurrent gene fusions have also been observed in solid cancers. In a study conducted by Pan T et al., 2020, they have identified around 11 fused genes in OSCC, in which one of them is involved in OSCC progression. They found that the gene fusion Tripartite Motif Containing 52 - Receptor For Activated C Kinase 1 (TRIM52-RACK1) was caused by a deletion of 181,257,187-181,247,386 at 5q35.3 and it induces OSCC cell proliferation, migration and invasion (Pan et al. 2020). Some other similar studies also have detected gene fusions in OSCC which facilitates carcinogenesis and aggressiveness (Guo et al. 2016), (N. Singh et al. 2020). In addition, gene fusions are also reported in other types of cancers such as in prostate cancer, where a serine protease gene, androgen-regulated trans-membrane protease, serine 2 (TMPRSS2) was found to be fused with either Erythroblast Transformation Specific related gene (ERG) or ETS Variant Transcription Factor 1 (ETV1), which are members of the ETS family of oncogenes (Narod, Seth, and Nam 2008). Tomlins et al., 2005 reported that out of the 29 prostate cancer samples that were studied, 23 contained TMPRSS2-ERG or TMPRSS2-ETV1 fusion (Tomlins et al. 2005). In high-grade serous ovarian cancer (HGSC), a gene fusion between Basal Cell Adhesion Molecule (BCAM) which is a membrane adhesion molecule, and AKT Serine/Threonine Kinase 2 (AKT2), a key kinase in the PI3K signalling pathway was also observed. In non-small cell lung cancers (NSCLC) patients, echinoderm microtubule-associated protein-like 4 and anaplastic lymphoma kinase (EML4-ALK) fusions have been observed (Koivunen et al. 2008). Classifying the subtypes of cancer based on these recurrent gene fusions can also aid in the treatment of the disease. For example, in NSCLC patients, who have the EML4-ALK fusion gene, ALK inhibitor alone or in combination with other kinase inhibitors could be used as an effective treatment (Koivunen et al. 2008).

Deletion is another chromosomal rearrangement that has been shown to play a major role in the development and progression of cancer where deletion of chromosomal regions may lead to the loss of certain tumour suppressor genes. Identifying these deletions may have remarkable significance in determining disease outcomes such as lymph node metastasis. These molecular classifications may also help in the early prediction of the disease or treatments such as personalised medicine. Deletions of a region in a chromosome or of a particular gene has been reported in several cancers. In a study conducted by Sukhija H et al., 2015 it has been revealed that out of 20 OSCC patient samples collected, each sample has a C- deletion mutation in exon 4 codon 63 of the p53 gene (Sukhija et al. 2015). The deletion of the gene GSTT1 which codes for Glutathione S-transferase Theta-1 enzyme has been observed to promote the risk of OSCC development (Neves Drummond et al. 2005). In addition, the deletion of phosphatase and tensin homolog (PTEN), a tumour suppressor gene was seen in 68% of samples of prostate cancer patients (Yoshimoto et al. 2006). In a study done on 38 NSCLC patients, two genes Hyaluronidase-2 (HYAL2) and Fragile Histidine Triad Protein (FHIT) were observed to be deleted in 84% and 79% tumours respectively. It was also reported that 54% of patients who had HYAL2 deletions in tumour tissues also showed such deletions in their sputum and 50% of patients with FHIT deletions in tumours had the same deletion in their sputum. Therefore, HYAL2 and FHIT deletions in sputum may be used as diagnostic biomarkers for early-stage lung cancers (Vincent-Chong et al. 2017) In OSCC, deletions in 3p and 8p chromosomal regions, specifically at 3p21.31, 3p26.3-p26.1 and 8p23.2 were observed to be recurrent (Vincent-Chong et al. 2017). The genetic alteration in OSCC by combining array-based comparative genomic hybridization and multiplex ligation-dependent probe amplification technique was best studied by Cha et al., 2011. This study revealed that many of the genes such as Family with Sequence Similarity 5, Member B (FAM5B), Tetrachlorodibenzo-p-dioxin (TCDD)-inducible poly (ADP-ribose) polymerase (TiPARP), Phosphatidylinositol-4,5-Bisphosphate 3-Kinase Catalytic Subunit Alpha (PIK3CA), Neuroligin 1 (NLGN1), Fibroblast Growth Factor 10 (FGF10), Histone Deacetylase 9 (HDAC9), Glutamate Metabotropic Receptor 3 (GRM3), Development And Differentiation Enhancing Factor 1 (DDEF1), Endothelin Receptor Type B (EDNRB), Chordin Like 1 (CHRDL1), and 5-Hydroxytryptamine Receptor

2C (HTR2C) are amplified and genes such as Thyroid Hormone Receptor Associated Protein 3 (THRAP3), Cortactin Binding Protein 2 N-terminal-like Protein (CTTNBP2NL), GATA Zinc Finger Domain Containing 2B (GATAD2B), REL, Cytoskeleton Associated Protein 2 Like (CKAP2L), Ras Homolog Family Member A (RHOA), Eukaryotic Translation Initiation Factor 4E Family Member 3 (EIF4E3), PDZ And LIM Domain 5 (PDLIM5), F-Box Protein 3 (FBXO3), Neuronal Differentiation 4 (NEUROD4), and ATP Binding Cassette Subfamily A Member 5 (ABCA5) are deleted during the progression of OSCC (Cha, Kim, and Cha 2011).

Detection of these chromosomal rearrangements is of utmost importance as they play an important role as biomarkers. Fluorescence in situ hybridization which has been used as the gold standard for detecting structural chromosomal rearrangements has been shown to have a limited resolution and often needs to be substantiated by some other method or cytogenetic technique to increase resolution and provide accurate results. Mate pair whole genome sequencing (MP-WGS) is a technique that has been used to accompany karyotype analysis to detect structural chromosomal rearrangements. When MP-WGS was used to sequence ten bone marrow samples from leukaemia patients with recurrent rearrangements, all the rearrangements that were identified by FISH were successfully detected. MP-WGS also revealed additional rearrangements that were missed out by previous cytogenetic analysis. Coordinates for all detected rearrangement breakpoints were also identifiable using MP-WGS (Tran et al. 2018). When used for the characterisation of multiple myeloma, MP-WGS was observed to be a better method in identifying chromosomal rearrangements. Out of the 30 discordance cases between FISH analysis and MP-WGS, FISH analysis missed abnormalities in 19 cases which were identifiable using MP-WGS (Smadbeck et al. 2019).

EPIGENETIC MODIFICATIONS AS BIOMARKERS

Epigenetic changes refer to modifications that lead to the dysregulation of gene expression without altering the DNA sequence. Without changing the DNA sequence, these modifications are capable of turning genes "on" and "off" thus affecting their expression pattern. Epigenetic modifications regulate gene expression through two mechanisms:

1) *via* modifications on histone proteins that affect the tertiary structure of DNA, thus interfering with DNA-protein interactions, or
2) By directly causing modifications on the DNA strand itself

Modifications such as DNA methylation or histone acetylation/ methylations have been shown to cause changes in the process of chromatin condensation, thus affecting how transcription factors bind to promoter regions. Both DNA methylation and histone modifications are responsible for the altered gene expression that is observed in many human diseases including cancer.

Changes in DNA methylation observed in cancer has been an indication that it could be used as a target for developing biomarkers for diagnostic, prognostic and predictive purposes. Changes in DNA methylation patterns have been described in numerous cancers and it has been observed that these modifications are considered to be among the earliest aberrations that occur during carcinogenesis. The usage of several methylated genes as tumour biomarkers have been proposed for various cancers including breast (Obaidul et al. 2006; Kim et al. 2010; Kloten et al. 2013), lung (Vinayanuwattikun et al. 2011; Balgkouranidou et al. 2016; Powrózek et al. 2016), prostate (Payne et al. 2009; T. Wu et al. 2011; Haldrup et al. 2018) and gastric cancer (J. Nakamura et al. 2014; d'Errico et al. 2020; C. Li et al. 2020). In OSCC studies, promoter methylation of cell adhesion genes (Hsiao Wen Chang et al. 2002; Q. Chen et al. 2004; Mishra et al. 2018), cell-cycle control genes (Viswanathan, Tsuchida, and Shanmugam 2003; Strzelczyk, Krakowczyk, and Owczarek 2018; Allameh et al. 2019), apoptosis-related genes (Y. K. Wong, Lee, and Liu 2011; Y. Liu et al. 2012) and DNA-repair genes (Jayaprakash et al. 2017; Taioli et al. 2009; González-Ramírez et al. 2011; Czerninski et al. 2009) have been reported. Obtaining samples of plasma, serum, saliva and urine for the detection and analysis of these DNA methylation changes can be done in non-invasive or minimally invasive methods *via* liquid biopsies. Due to advancements in technology, currently there are numerous methods for identifying and measuring DNA methylation (Tost 2018). Methylation-specific polymerase chain reaction (MS-PCR) has been the most commonly adopted technique for determining promoter methylation levels in many cancer-related studies. MS-PCR is the preferred method as it provides rapid detection of the methylation status of the CpG islands, requires minute amounts of DNA, has high detection sensitivity and can be used for detecting methylation in different samples such as biofluids and even paraffin-embedded samples (Ramalho-Carvalho, Henrique, and Jerónimo 2018). The first part of this method is known as sodium bisulfite conversion, where unmethylated cytosines are converted to uracil and methylated cytosines remain unchanged. The converted sequence is then used as a template for PCR where primers and probes specific for the methylated and unmethylated sequences are used for quantitative analysis (Ramalho-Carvalho, Henrique, and Jerónimo 2018).

In eukaryotes, DNA in the nucleus is associated with certain proteins known as histone proteins forming a highly condense and a compact structure called chromatin. Histone methylation and acetylation/ deacetylation are factors that have been known to alter the structure of chromatin, thus influencing its function. Histone acetylation is usually associated with transcriptionally active genes, whereas the effect of methylation mainly depends on the number of methyl groups, the residue itself and its location within the histone tails. The enzymes involved in the processes of histone modifications include histone acetyltransferases (HATs), histone deacetylases (HDACs), histone methyltransferases (HMTs) and histone demethylases (HDMs). Numerous studies have reported that histone modifications can be used for the prognosis of cancer. Association between histone modification patterns and cancer detection, prognosis, recurrence and patient survival have been well explored in several cancers including lung (J. S. Song et al. 2012), prostate (Ellinger et al. 2010), breast (Elsheikh et al. 2009), leukaemia (Müller-Tidow et al. 2010) and oesophagal (Tzao et al. 2009) cancers. Immunohistochemistry has been the method that has been used in most studies to detect histone marks in tissue samples. The altered activity of HDACs has also been associated with the progression of several human cancers including lung (Osada et al. 2004; Sasaki et al. 2004), gastric (Weichert, Röske, Niesporek, et al. 2008; Weichert, Röske, Gekeler, et al. 2008) and prostate (Abbas and Gupta, n.d.) cancers. Several papers have also discussed the dysregulation of specific HDACs in OSCC. The overexpression of histone deacetylase 2 (HDAC2) (H. H. Chang et al. 2009) and histone deacetylase 6 (HDAC6) was observed in both OSCC cell lines and OSCC tissue samples as compared to normal oral keratinocytes and normal oral tissues. Significant differences in expression levels between the early stages and late stages of cancer also seems to suggest an association between HDAC6 expression levels and the clinical tumour stages, and overexpression of HDAC6 is observed in the later stages of OSCC (Sakuma et al. 2006). With further research into understanding how the dysregulation of these HDACs can be used as potential biomarkers for cancer and OSCC, new diagnostic and prognostic biomarkers could be developed.

RNA as Biomarkers

The potential use of RNAs as biomarkers for various cancers have been well explored and described in a multitude of papers (B. Yang et al. 2016; Hamam et al. 2017; S. wei Huang et al. 2018; G. Li et al. 2019; H. Liu et al. 2019). Information such as cellular stages and regulatory processes which cannot be obtained using DNA biomarkers can be obtained using RNA biomarkers. The variation in RNA copy numbers has also been shown to be a useful diagnostic tool to determine if a particular gene is being up or downregulated. The high sensitivity and specificity of RNA biomarkers allow even small traces of RNA to be amplified and captured using PCR. Using RNA biomarkers is also a cheaper alternative to protein biomarkers as detection of each protein requires a specific antibody. RNA dysregulation, specifically microRNAs (miRNA) dysregulation has been observed in different diseases including cancer, cardiovascular diseases (Akodad, Mericskay, and Roubille 2016; S. S. Zhou et al. 2018) and neurodegenerative diseases (Juźwik et al. 2019; Catanesi et al. 2020). There have been a multitude of papers that have described the alteration in miRNA expression in hepatocellular carcinoma (C. Peng et al. 2019), breast (Kashyap and Kaur 2020), lung (C. Hu et al. 2020), gastric (Stojanovic et al. 2019) and prostate (C. J. Song et al. 2018) cancers.

In addition to identifying tissue-based RNA biomarkers for diagnosis, there has been a great interest in identifying extracellular RNAs (exRNAs) as biomarkers due to the promising potential of developing a non-invasive diagnostic tool. ExRNAs are RNA molecules that are present outside the cells in which they were transcribed and can be found in biofluids such as whole blood, plasma, serum, urine, breast milk, saliva and cerebrospinal fluid. They are the signalling molecules that play a role in cell-cell communications (Dinger, Mercer, and Mattick 2008; Valadi et al. 2007) and are released by both normal cells and tumour cells but the differential expression of RNA from tumour cells can be of significant clinical relevance (Schwarzenbach et al. 2014). These exRNAs can be beneficial for the diagnosis and classification of cancers, especially when it might be difficult to obtain tumour tissues. The easiest method of obtaining exRNAs are through liquid biopsies which is a process of collecting body fluids to obtain diagnostic or prognostic information. Blood and saliva being the two most accessible biofluids are the most widely studied for determining and developing biomarkers.

miRNAs are the most widely studied mRNAs which showed promising results as cancer biomarkers. miRNAs are small, single-stranded, non-coding RNAs of approximately 22 nucleotides. They play a role in regulating the expression pattern of coding genes by interacting with their complementary sequences usually present in the 3′ untranslated regions (UTRs) of their target mRNAs.(Lewis et al. 2003) As miRNAs are involved in cell-cell communications, it has been established that miRNAs are expressed in a cell-specific manner, meaning that any regulatory changes or disease status in a cell will change the expression of miRNAs (Williams 2008) and due to their high tissue specificity, miRNAs are effective biomarkers for determining the tissue of origin in cancers (Rosenfeld et al. 2008). Due to their small size, as compared to mRNAs, miRNAs are more stable allowing for easier expression profiling from biological materials and thus promoting their use as non-invasive biomarkers. Some miRNAs are upregulated, implicating their role as oncogenes whereas some miRNAs have been reported to be downregulated thus demonstrating tumour suppressive roles in OSCC tumorigenesis. Some reports have shown that dysregulated miRNA levels return to relatively normal levels after tumour resection and treatments such as chemotherapy. Sun et al., reported that the high levels of serum miR-155 in breast cancer patients are significantly reduced, reaching levels comparable to those of the controls, after tumour resection and chemotherapy. This trend of declined serum miRNA levels in post-operative samples were also observed in lung carcinoma (Le et al. 2012), renal cell carcinoma (X. Chen et al. 2018), colorectal cancer (Y. Zhao, Ren, and Zhu 2018) and oral squamous cell carcinoma (OSCC) (Romani et al. 2021). These studies provide evidences of the correlation between serum and salivary miRNA levels and tumour dynamics. The development of miRNA biomarker panels for OSCC diagnosis has also been studied by few groups. Biomarker panels have been shown to demonstrate a higher diagnostic power as compared to a single miRNA. Nakamura et al., 2021 concluded that a combination of 6 differently expressed miRNAs, namely, miR-24, miR-20a, miR-122, miR-150, miR-4419a and miR-5100 were capable of diagnosing OSCC by significantly distinguishing the expression between OSCC samples and healthy controls with a high degree of accuracy (K. Nakamura et al. 2021). Another group studied a cohort of two hundred and fifty Taiwanese patients and identified 3 plasma miRNAs for the detection of OSCC. The miRNA panel consisting of miR-222-3p, miR-150-5p and miR-423-5p were shown to be effective for early detection of OSCC (Y. A. Chang et al. 2018).

Analysing mRNA expression levels is one of the easiest ways to study gene expression, and therefore, there have been many studies that have reported the prospective mRNA biomarkers that can be used for cancer detection, diagnosis and prognosis. As many genes are dysregulated in cancer, a multitude of papers have described the various mRNAs that are involved in different cancers. Studies have shown that circulating cell-free mRNA present in biofluids such as blood and saliva can be used as tumour markers. The diagnostic and prognostic value of such mRNAs have been tested in several cancers including gastric cancer (TANI et al. 2007; C. Su et al. 2019), breast cancer (Yanlin Wu et al. 2018; Ma et al. 2019), lung cancer (S. Karimi et al. 2015) and OSCC (Elashoff et al. 2006; Márton et al. 2019; St. John et al. 2004; Hsueh Wei Chang et al. 2018; Oh et al. 2020).

Circular RNAs (circRNAs) are a group of non-coding RNAs which have a covalently closed circular structure with transcript lengths of hundreds to thousands of nucleotides. Due to their circular structure, circRNAs have an increased resistance to digestion by exonucleases and therefore gets accumulated in tissues and body fluids. The expression of circRNAs is tissue-specific and recent studies have reported that circRNAs are also differentially expressed in several human tumours. The potential of using circRNAs as biomarkers for the diagnosis and prognosis of cancer as well as for monitoring treatment response have been studied. Studies showing the promising use of circRNAs as biomarkers have been demonstrated in gastric cancer (P. Li et al. 2015; Shao et al. 2017), lung cancer (J. T. Yao et al. 2017; Tan et al. 2018), colorectal cancer (W. Weng et al. 2017; J. Lin et al. 2019) and hepatocellular carcinoma (Yu et al. 2016; L. Fu et al. 2017). The upregulation of hsa_circ_0001874, hsa_circ_0001971 and hsa_circ_0008068 and the downregulation of hsa_circ_0000140, hsa_circ_0002632 and hsa_circ_0008792 in saliva has been observed in OSCC patients (S.-Y. Zhao et al. 2018).

Long noncoding RNAs (lncRNAs) are a group of RNAs that have transcripts ranging from 200 nucleotides to 100 kb. When first identified, lncRNAs were initially thought to be a by-product of transcription with practically no or very little function. However, subsequent studies revealed the possible role that lncRNAs play in various cellular processes including cell growth, cell differentiation, cell fate determination and even apoptosis (W. Hu, Alvarez-Dominguez, and Lodish 2012; Flynn and Chang 2014; Rossi and Antonangeli 2014). The dysregulation of lncRNAs has also been observed in cancers and studies have revealed how lncRNAs play a role in regulating cancer cell proliferation, invasion and migration (B. Liu et al. 2016; Qian et al. 2017; Z. Y. Yang et al. 2017).

Table 3. The different types of RNA used as a biomarker and its type of regulation in Oral Squamous Cell Carcinoma

Types of RNA		Sources	Regulation	Sample sizes		References
				Cases	Control	
miRNA	miR-21	Blood	Upregulated	58	32	(Ren et al. 2014)
		Serum	Upregulated	20	40	(P. Singh et al. 2018)
		Serum	Upregulated	20	20	(A. Karimi et al. 2020)
		Plasma	Upregulated	100	100	(Mahmood et al. 2019)
	miR-24	Saliva	Upregulated	45	10	(He et al. 2020)
		Tissue	Upregulated	43	43	(S. C. Lin et al. 2010)
		Plasma	Upregulated	33	10	(S. C. Lin et al. 2010)
	miR-31	Saliva	Upregulated	45	24	(Chung Ji Liu et al. 2012)
		Saliva	Upregulated	35	20	(Kadhim Al-Malkey et al. 2015)
		Plasma	Upregulated	43	21	(C. J. Liu et al. 2010)
		Tissue	Upregulated	51	40	(Lajer et al. 2011)
	miR-200b	Plasma	Upregulated	80	80	(G. Sun et al. 2018)
	miR-483-5p	Serum	Upregulated	101	103	(H. Xu et al. 2016)
		Tissue (esophageal squamous cell carcinoma)	Upregulated	80	80	(Xue et al. 2017)

Types of RNA		Sources	Regulation	Sample sizes		References
				Cases	Control	
	miR-184	Tissue (tongue squamous cell carcinoma)	Upregulated	50	50	(Ghaffari et al. 2020)
		Plasma (tongue squamous cell carcinoma)	Upregulated	30	38	(T. S. Wong et al. 2008)
	miR-27a	Tissue	Downregulated	50	50	(G. Zeng et al. 2016)
	miR-99a	Tissue	Downregulated	40	40	(Yen et al. 2014)
		Serum	Downregulated	121	55	(L. Chen et al. 2018)
	miR-138	Tissue	Downregulated	20	20	(R. Xu et al. 2015)
		Tissue	Downregulated	254	4	(D. Zeng et al. 2019)
	miR-145	Tissue	Downregulated	62	62	(Gao et al. 2013)
		Saliva	Downregulated	20	20	(Zahran et al. 2015)
	miR-375	Tissue	Downregulated	26	3	(Siow et al. 2014)
		Tissue	Downregulated	51	40	(Lajer et al. 2011)
		Plasma	Downregulated	20	18	(Yan et al. 2017)
mRNA	Ras homolog gene family, member A *(ARCR)*	Serum	Upregulated	32	35	(Elashoff et al. 2006)
	Ferritin, heavy polypeptide 1 *(FTH1)*	Serum	Upregulated	32	35	(Elashoff et al. 2006)
	H3 histone, family 3A *(H3F3A)*	Serum	Upregulated	32	35	(Elashoff et al. 2006)
	IL-6	Saliva	Upregulated	95	80	(Márton et al. 2019)
		Saliva	Upregulated	32	32	(St. John et al. 2004)
	IL-8	Saliva	Upregulated	32	32	(St. John et al. 2004)
	Integrin Subunit Alpha 3 (ITGA3)	Tissue	Upregulated	55	55	(Hsueh Wei Chang et al. 2018)

Table 3. (Continued)

Types of RNA		Sources	Regulation	Sample sizes		References
				Cases	Control	
	Integrin Subunit Alpha 5 (ITGA5)	Tissue	Upregulated	55	55	(Hsueh Wei Chang et al. 2018)
	Integrin Subunit Beta 1 (ITGB1)	Tissue	Upregulated	55	55	(Hsueh Wei Chang et al. 2018)
	Integrin Subunit Beta 6 (ITGB6)	Tissue	Upregulated	55	55	(Hsueh Wei Chang et al. 2018)
	Nuclear Receptor Coactivator 4 (NCOA4)	Serum	Upregulated	32	35	(Elashoff et al. 2006)
	Tumor Protein, Translationally-Controlled 1 (TPT1)	Serum	Upregulated	32	35	(Elashoff et al. 2006)
	Monoamine Oxidase B (MAOB)	Saliva	Downregulated	33	34	(Oh et al. 2020)
	NGFI-A Binding Protein 2 (NAB2)	Saliva	Downregulated	33	34	(Oh et al. 2020)
	Collagen, Type III, Alpha 1 (COL3A1)	Saliva	Downregulated	33	34	(Oh et al. 2020)
	Cytochrome P450, Family 27, Subfamily A, Polypeptide 1 (CYP27A1)	Saliva	Downregulated	33	34	(Oh et al. 2020)
	Nuclear Pore Complex Interacting Protein Family, Member B4 (NPIPB4)	Saliva	Downregulated	33	34	(Oh et al. 2020)
	Sialic Acid Acetyltransferase (SIAE)	Saliva	Downregulated	33	34	(Oh et al. 2020)
circRNAs	hsa_circ_0001874	Saliva	Upregulated	93	85	(S.-Y. Zhao et al. 2018)
	hsa_circ_0001971	Saliva	Upregulated	93	85	(S.-Y. Zhao et al. 2018)

Types of RNA		Sources	Regulation	Sample sizes		References
				Cases	Control	
	hsa_circ_0008068	Saliva	Upregulated	93	85	(S.-Y. Zhao et al. 2018)
	hsa_circ_0000140	Saliva	Downregulated	93	85	(S.-Y. Zhao et al. 2018)
	hsa_circ_0002632	Saliva	Downregulated	93	85	(S.-Y. Zhao et al. 2018)
	hsa_circ_0008309	Tissue	Downregulated	45	45	(B. Li et al. 2018)
	hsa_circ_0008792	Saliva	Downregulated	93	85	(S.-Y. Zhao et al. 2018)
	hsa_circ_001242	Tissue	Downregulated	40	40	(S. Sun et al. 2018)
	hsa_circ_0072387	Tissue	Downregulated	63	63	(Dou et al. 2019)
	hsa_circ_0086414	Tissue	Downregulated	55	55	(L. Li and Zhang 2020)
	hsa_circ_009755	Tissue	Downregulated	8	8	(Zhang et al. 2020)
		Tissue	Downregulated	27	27	(Z. Wang et al. 2019)
lncRNAs	HOX Antisense Intergenic RNA (HOTAIR)	Tissue	Upregulated	4	4	(H. Tang et al. 2013)
		Tissue	Upregulated	76	76	(Yansheng Wu et al. 2015)
	Highly Up-Regulated In Liver Cancer (HULC)	Tissue	Upregulated	4	4	(H. Tang et al. 2013)
	Nuclear Paraspeckle Assembly Transcript 1 (NEAT-1)	Tissue	Upregulated	4	4	(H. Tang et al. 2013)
	Urothelial Cancer Associated 1 (UCA1)	Tissue	Upregulated	4	4	(H. Tang et al. 2013)
		Tissue (tongue squamous cell carcinoma)	Upregulated	94	94	(Fang et al. 2014)
	U62317.1	Tissue	Upregulated	167	45	(Y. Li, Cao, and Li 2020)
	Maternally Expressed 3 (MEG-3)	Tissue	Downregulated	4	4	(H. Tang et al. 2013)

Table 3. (Continued)

Types of RNA		Sources	Regulation	Sample sizes		References
				Cases	Control	
	Long Intergenic Non-Protein Coding RNA 1697 (LINC01697)	Tissue	Downregulated	167	45	(Y. Li, Cao, and Li 2020)
	Long Intergenic Non-Protein Coding RNA 2487 (LINC02487)	Tissue	Downregulated	167	45	(Y. Li, Cao, and Li 2020)
	LOC105376575	Tissue	Downregulated	167	45	(Y. Li, Cao, and Li 2020)
	AC005083.1	Tissue	Downregulated	167	45	(Y. Li, Cao, and Li 2020)
	Solute Carrier Family 8 Member A1 Antisense RNA 1 (SLC8A1-AS1)	Tissue	Downregulated	167	45	(Y. Li, Cao, and Li 2020)

The usage of lncRNAs as biomarkers for the diagnosis and prognosis of cancer has been reported in oesophagal cancer (Tong et al. 2015; W. Wang et al. 2017), gastric cancer (Pang et al. 2014; Shao et al. 2014), hepatocellular carcinoma (J. Tang et al. 2015; T. Zhou and Gao 2016) and colorectal cancer (Ge et al. 2013; Svoboda et al. 2014). In OSCC, HOX Antisense Intergenic RNA (HOTAIR), Nuclear Paraspeckle Assembly Transcript 1 (NEAT-1), Highly Up-Regulated In Liver Cancer (HULC) and Urothelial Cancer Associated 1 (UCA1) are some of the lncRNAs that have been reported to be upregulated (H. Tang et al. 2013; Yansheng Wu et al. 2015). One of the main advantages of lncRNAs that make them suitable for usage of biomarkers is their high stability and resistance to ribonucleases when present in body fluids. Additionally, the lncRNA deregulation observed in primary tumour tissues have been shown to be the same in body fluids including blood, plasma, serum, saliva and urine. These characteristics of lncRNAs provide a promising opportunity for developing beneficial and minimally invasive biomarkers for cancer. The different types of RNA biomarkers implicated in OSCC is shown in Table 3.

Proteomic Biomarkers

As the development and progression of cancer are driven by changes in the dysregulation of a variety of genes that are involved in cell proliferation, differentiation and death, it is evident that there must be changes in the expression levels of numerous proteins as well. These changes in protein expression levels might lead to changes in cell growth, metabolism and even affect cell signalling. It has been shown that certain tumour-specific proteins produced by cancer cells may enter the patient's circulation and these proteins can act as diagnostic or prognostic cancer biomarkers (Tung et al. 2013; Núñez 2019; El-Khoury et al. 2020). Protein-based biomarkers have been identified in several cancers including hepatocellular carcinoma (Waidely et al. 2016), lung cancer (Zamay et al. 2017), colorectal cancer (Wilhelmsen et al. 2017), pancreatic cancer (Cohen et al. 2017) and OSCC. In a study done on 48 OSCC patients and 48 controls, five candidate biomarkers, Human Mac-2 binding protein (M2BP), Migration inhibitory factor-related protein 14 (MRP14), CD59, catalase and profilin were observed to be differently expressed in saliva with the potential of being OSCC biomarkers (S. Hu et al. 2008). In another study, five other proteins in saliva, Complement Factor B (CFB), Complement C3 (C3), Complement C4B (C4B), serine protease inhibitor Family A Member 1 (SERPINA1) and Leucine-Rich Alpha-2-Glycoprotein 1 (LRG1) were shown to be candidate biomarkers for OSCC (Kawahara et al. 2016). Serum-based proteomic biomarkers have also been studied and identified in OSCC (Bijian et al. 2009; Y. Yang et al. 2014). Chai et al., 2016 reported that four serum protein biomarkers, namely, gelsolin, fibronectin, angiotensinogen and haptoglobin were shown to be differentially expressed between node-positive and node-negative cancer cell lines, indicating that identification of the biomarkers could be used for the prediction of metastasis in OSCC (Chai et al. 2016). Proteomic based identification of tumour biomarkers can be done using several techniques such as 2D gel electrophoresis, mass spectrometry, liquid chromatography coupled to mass spectrometry (LCMS) and more recently, matrix assist laser desorption ionization (MALDI)-based imaging of tissues (Maruvada et al. 2005).

Metabolomic Biomarkers

Metabolomic biomarkers in OSCC include carbohydrates, enzymes, metabolites and liquid biomarkers. During OSCC progression, the alterations in the expression of O-linked and N-linked glycans occur. These altered carbohydrate markers can be used as an influential biomarkers for OSCC detection. These markers from human samples such as serum, cancer cell lines or tissues obtained from biopsies are profiled using MALDI-TOF, Electrospray Ionization (ESI) etc., The most frequently used techniques to analyze metabolomic biomarkers in cancer are by Mass-Spectrometry (MS), Liquid Chromatography, Nuclear Magnetic Resonance, enzyme assays etc., (Arglebe 1981). The glycomarkers such as glycoproteins, proteoglycans, glycolipids are more stable than RNA and proteins. These markers are reported to be ideal for cancer prediction studies where screening of samples for the probability of carcinogenesis in the future can be analysed. It is reported that in many types of cancers, there are modifications in the glycomarkers as cancer progresses and these can be used to identify carcinogenesis (Saldova et al. 2008; Powlesland et al. 2009; Misonou et al. 2009; Abbott et al. 2008).

Challenges in OSCC Biomarker Development

Few challenges faced by researchers in developing clinical cancer biomarkers are (i) the preparation of the sample is non-uniform, (ii) the difficulty in the storage of the sample, (iii) some techniques gives enormous data which makes it difficult to analyze, and (iv) cancer tissues comprise of disorganized cells as a result of mutations and all these limitations are challenges associated with biomarker development. In malignant conditions, the inherited genetic instability could pave the way to the new tumour cell subpopulation which can expand quickly as the growth potential increases (Vadas et al. 2008). During OSCC progression, the emergence of new clones with genetic and epigenetic alterations occurs, termed as “clonal diversity,” which happens as a result of mutations and structural alterations. The clonal diversity along with genetic, epigenetic, heterogeneous nature of cells, histological aberrations increases with ageing that additionally complicates the detection of OSCC. As a result, many biomarkers may not even express during the detection process. Other problems are because of the over-detection, non-specific binding and over-treatment strategies of biomarkers resulting in misinterpretation of cancers including OSCC.

CONCLUSION

To reduce the impediments associated with the use of biomarkers based detection of OSCC, it is crucial to understand the types, steps and protocol of application of the biomarkers to evaluate the appropriate biomarkers according to the types and stages of the tumour. Further research should focus on developing new biomarkers for a heterogeneous population of cancer cells and its host-immune response. Distinct studies should be conducted on the diagnostic biomarkers and therapeutic targets. Accordingly, the mechanism of OSCC oncogenesis has to be studied in detail for the identification of a reliable gene that could be used as a biomarker to predict the possibilities of OSCC occurrence and to prevent the advancement of OSCC. To reduce the patient mortality and morbidity rate of OSCC, it is highly suggested to develop valid clinical candidate markers with high clinical utility and screening efficacy.

REFERENCES

Abbas, Ata, and Sanjay Gupta. n.d. "The Role of Histone Deacetylases in Prostate Cancer." *Epigenetics* 3 (6): 300–309. https://doi.org/10.4161/epi.3.6.7273.

Abbott, Karen L., Alison V. Nairn, Erica M. Hall, Marc B. Horton, John F. McDonald, Kelley W. Moremen, Daniela M. Dinulescu, and Michael

Pierce. 2008. "Focused Glycomic Analysis of the N-Linked Glycan Biosynthetic Pathway in Ovarian Cancer." *Proteomics* 8 (16): 3210–20. https://doi.org/10.1002/pmic.200800157.

Akodad, Mariama, Mathias Mericskay, and François Roubille. 2016. "Micro-RNAs as Promising Biomarkers in Cardiac Diseases." *Annals of Translational Medicine*. AME Publishing Company. https://doi.org/10.21037/atm.2016.12.38.

Allameh, Abdolamir, Abdolkarim Moazeni-Roodi, Iraj Harirchi, Mehrdad Ravanshad, Maziar Motiee-Langroudi, Ata Garajei, Azin Hamidavi, and Seyed Alireza Mesbah-Namin. 2019. "Promoter DNA Methylation and MRNA Expression Level of P16 Gene in Oral Squamous Cell Carcinoma: Correlation with Clinicopathological Characteristics." *Pathology and Oncology Research* 25 (4): 1535–43. https://doi.org/10.1007/s12253-018-0542-1.

Allegra, Carmen J., J. Milburn Jessup, Mark R. Somerfield, Stanley R. Hamilton, Elizabeth H. Hammond, Daniel F. Hayes, Pamela K. McAllister, Roscoe F. Morton, and Richard L. Schilsky. 2009. "American Society of Clinical Oncology Provisional Clinical Opinion: Testing for KRAS Gene Mutations in Patients with Metastatic Colorectal Carcinoma to Predict Response to Anti-Epidermal Growth Factor Receptor Monoclonal Antibody Therapy." *Journal of Clinical Oncology* 27 (12): 2091–96. https://doi.org/10.1200/JCO.2009.21.9170.

Arglebe, C. 1981. "Biochemistry of Human Saliva." *Advances in Oto-Rhino-Laryngology* 26: 97–234. https://doi.org/10.1159/000395291.

Azevedo, Ana P., Susana N. Silva, Alice Reichert, Fernando Lima, Esmeraldina Júnior, and José Rueff. 2019. "The Role of Caspase Genes Polymorphisms in Genetic Susceptibility to Philadelphia-Negative Myeloproliferative Neoplasms in a Portuguese Population." *Pathology and Oncology Research* 25 (3): 961–69. https://doi.org/10.1007/s12253-018-0411-y.

Babji, Deepa, Ramakant Nayak, Kishore Bhat, and Vijayalakshmi Kotrashetti. 2019. "Cell-Free Tumor DNA: Emerging Reality in Oral Squamous Cell Carcinoma." *Journal of Oral and Maxillofacial*

Pathology 23 (2): 273–79. https://doi.org/10.4103/jomfp.JOMFP_36_19.

Bagán, José V., Judith Murillo, Rafael Poveda, Carmen Gavaldá, Yolanda Jiménez, and Crispian Scully. 2004. "Proliferative Verrucous Leukoplakia: Unusual Locations of Oral Squamous Cell Carcinomas, and Field Cancerization as Shown by the Appearance of Multiple OSCCs." *Oral Oncology* 40 (4): 440–43. https://doi.org/10.1016/j.oraloncology.2003.10.008.

Balgkouranidou, Ioanna, Maria Chimonidou, Georgia Milaki, Emily Tsaroucha, Stylianos Kakolyris, Vasilis Georgoulias, and Evi Lianidou. 2016. "SOX17 Promoter Methylation in Plasma Circulating Tumor DNA of Patients with Non-Small Cell Lung Cancer." *Clinical Chemistry and Laboratory Medicine* 54 (8): 1385–93. https://doi.org/10.1515/cclm-2015-0776.

Ballman, Karla V. 2015. "Biomarker: Predictive or Prognostic?" *Journal of Clinical Oncology* 33 (33): 3968–71. https://doi.org/10.1200/JCO.2015.63.3651.

Bánóczy, J. 1997. "Oral Cancer and Precancerous Lesions." *Fogorvosi Szemle* 90 Spec No: 27. https://doi.org/10.3322/canjclin.52.4.195.

Bettegowda C., Sausen M., Leary R. J., Kinde I., Wang Y., Agrawal N., Bartlett B. R., Wang H., Luber B., Alani R. M., Antonarakis E. S. n.d. *Detection of Circulating Tumor DNA in Early-and Late-Stage Human Malignancies.*

Bewley, Arnaud F., and D. Gregory Farwell. 2017. "Oral Leukoplakia and Oral Cavity Squamous Cell Carcinoma." *Clinics in Dermatology* 35 (5): 461–67. https://doi.org/10.1016/j.clindermatol.2017.06.008.

Bhalang, Kanokporn, Anocha Suesuwan, Kittipong Dhanuthai, Phakdee Sannikorn, Lakana Luangjarmekorn, and Somporn Swasdison. 2008. "The Application of Acetic Acid in the Detection of Oral Squamous Cell Carcinoma." *Oral Surgery, Oral Medicine, Oral Pathology, Oral Radiology and Endodontology* 106 (3): 371–76. https://doi.org/10.1016/j.tripleo.2008.01.017.

Bhatia, Nirav, Yastira Lalla, An N. Vu, and Camile S. Farah. 2013. "Advances in Optical Adjunctive Aids for Visualisation and Detection of Oral Malignant and Potentially Malignant Lesions." *International Journal of Dentistry* 2013. https://doi.org/10.1155/2013/194029.

Bijian, Krikor, Alex M. Mlynarek, Richard L. Balys, Su Jie, Yingjie Xu, Michael P. Hier, Martin J. Black, Marcos R.Di Falco, Sylvie LaBoissiere, and Moulay A. Alaoui-Jamali. 2009. "Serum Proteomic Approach for the Identification of Serum Biomarkers Contributed by Oral Squamous Cell Carcinoma and Host Tissue Microenvironment." *Journal of Proteome Research* 8 (5): 2173–85. https://doi.org/10.1021/pr800979e.

Blatt, Sebastian, Maximilian Krüger, Thomas Ziebart, Keyvan Sagheb, Eik Schiegnitz, Elisabeth Goetze, Bilal Al-Nawas, and Andreas Max Pabst. 2017. "Biomarkers in Diagnosis and Therapy of Oral Squamous Cell Carcinoma: A Review of the Literature." *Journal of Cranio-Maxillofacial Surgery* 45 (5): 722–30. https://doi.org/10.1016/j.jcms.2017.01.033.

Bongiorno, Michelle, Shayna Rivard, Daniel Hammer, and Joshua Kentosh. 2017. "Malignant Transformation of Oral Leukoplakia in a Patient with Dyskeratosis Congenita." *Oral Surgery, Oral Medicine, Oral Pathology and Oral Radiology* 124 (4): e239–42. https://doi.org/10.1016/j.oooo.2017.08.001.

Borase, Archana P., Sindhu M. Ganvir, Vinay K. Hazarey, Suchitra R. Gosavi, Anand A. Mohatta, and Jasmine Singh. 2015. "Estimation of Vascular Endothelial Growth Factor Gene -460 C/T Polymorphism as a Biomarker in Oral Squamous Cell Carcinoma Patients from the Indian Subcontinent." *Journal of Investigative and Clinical Dentistry* 6 (4): 267–72. https://doi.org/10.1111/jicd.12103.

Braakhuis, B. J., Tabor, M. P., Kummer, J. A., Leemans, C. R., & Brakenhoff, R. H. n.d. *A Genetic Explanation of Slaughter's Concept of Field Cancerization: Evidence and Clinical Implications.*

Bremmer, Jantine F., Boudewijn J. M. Braakhuis, Henrique J. Ruijter-Schippers, Arjen Brink, Helena M.B. Duarte, Dirk J. Kuik, Elisabeth Bloemena, C. René Leemans, Isaäc Van Der Waal, and Ruud H. Brakenhoff. 2005. "A Noninvasive Genetic Screening Test to Detect

Oral Preneoplastic Lesions." *Laboratory Investigation* 85 (12): 1481–88. https://doi.org/10.1038/labinvest.3700342.

Cao, Zheng Guo, and Cheng Zhang Li. 2006. "A Single Nucleotide Polymorphism in the Matrix Metalloproteinase-1 Promoter Enhances Oral Squamous Cell Carcinoma Susceptibility in a Chinese Population." *Oral Oncology* 42 (1): 31–37. https://doi.org/10.1016/j.oraloncology.2004.08.015.

Catanesi, Mariano, Michele D'angelo, Maria Grazia Tupone, Elisabetta Benedetti, Antonio Giordano, Vanessa Castelli, and Annamaria Cimini. 2020. "Micrornas Dysregulation and Mitochondrial Dysfunction in Neurodegenerative Diseases." *International Journal of Molecular Sciences*. MDPI AG. https://doi.org/10.3390/ijms21175986.

Cha, Jeong Dan, Hyung Jun Kim, and In Ho Cha. 2011. "Genetic Alterations in Oral Squamous Cell Carcinoma Progression Detected by Combining Array-Based Comparative Genomic Hybridization and Multiplex Ligation-Dependent Probe Amplification." *Oral Surgery, Oral Medicine, Oral Pathology, Oral Radiology and Endodontology* 111 (5): 594–607. https://doi.org/10.1016/j.tripleo.2010.11.020.

Chai, Yang D., Lifeng Zhang, Yan Yang, Trent Su, Prashant Charugundla, Jiye Ai, Diana Messadi, David T. Wong, and Shen Hu. 2016. "Discovery of Potential Serum Protein Biomarkers for Lymph Node Metastasis in Oral Cancer." *Head and Neck* 38 (1): 118–25. https://doi.org/10.1002/hed.23870.

Chang, Hao Hueng, Chun Pin Chiang, Hsin Chia Hung, Chiao Ying Lin, Yi Ting Deng, and Mark Yen Ping Kuo. 2009. "Histone Deacetylase 2 Expression Predicts Poorer Prognosis in Oral Cancer Patients." *Oral Oncology* 45 (7): 610–14. https://doi.org/10.1016/j.oraloncology.2008.08.011.

Chang, Hsiao Wen, Vivian Chow, King Yin Lam, William Ignace Wei, and Anthony Po WingYuen. 2002. "Loss of E-Cadherin Expression Resulting from Promoter Hypermethylation in Oral Tongue Carcinoma and Its Prognostic Significance." *Cancer* 94 (2): 386–92. https://doi.org/10.1002/cncr.10211.

Chang, Hsueh Wei, Ching Yu Yen, Chung Ho Chen, Jun Hsu Tsai, Jen Yang Tang, Yung Ting Chang, Yu Hsun Kao, Yen Yun Wang, Shyng Shiou F. Yuan, and Sheng Yang Lee. 2018. "Evaluation of the MRNA Expression Levels of Integrins A3, A5, B1 and B6 as Tumor Biomarkers of Oral Squamous Cell Carcinoma." *Oncology Letters* 16 (4): 4773–81. https://doi.org/10.3892/ol.2018.9168.

Chang, Yi An, Shun Long Weng, Shun Fa Yang, Chih Hung Chou, Wei Chih Huang, Siang Jyun Tu, Tzu Hao Chang, Chien Ning Huang, Yuh Jyh Jong, and Hsien Da Huang. 2018. "A Three–MicroRNA Signature as a Potential Biomarker for the Early Detection of Oral Cancer." *International Journal of Molecular Sciences* 19 (3). https://doi.org/10.3390/ijms19030758.

Chen, Chu, Yuzheng Zhang, Melissa M. Loomis, Melissa P. Upton, Pawadee Lohavanichbutr, John R. Houck, David R. Doody, et al. 2015. "Genome-Wide Loss of Heterozygosity and DNA Copy Number Aberration in HPVNegative Oral Squamous Cell Carcinoma and Their Associations with Disease-Specific Survival." *PLoS ONE* 10 (8). https://doi.org/10.1371/journal.pone.0135074.

Chen, Liang, Jing Hu, Lina Pan, Xiaochun Yin, Qibao Wang, and Hui Chen. 2018. "Diagnostic and Prognostic Value of Serum MiR-99a Expression in Oral Squamous Cell Carcinoma." *Cancer Biomarkers* 23 (3): 333–39. https://doi.org/10.3233/CBM-181265.

Chen, Qianming, Galina Lipkina, Qi Song, and Randall H. Kramer. 2004. "Promoter Methylation Regulates Cadherin Switching in Squamous Cell Carcinoma." *Biochemical and Biophysical Research Communications* 315 (4): 850–56. https://doi.org/10.1016/j.bbrc.2004.01.143.

Chen, Xuanyu, Ning Lou, Anming Ruan, Bin Qiu, Yun Yan, Xuegang Wang, Quansheng Du, et al. 2018. "Mir-224/Mir-141 Ratio as a Novel Diagnostic Biomarker in Renal Cell Carcinoma." *Oncology Letters* 16 (2): 1666–74. https://doi.org/10.3892/ol.2018.8874.

Chen, Ya Wei, Jiun Sheng Lin, Cheng Hsien Wu, Man Tien Lui, Shou Yen Kao, and Yao Fong. 2007. "Application of in Vivo Stain of Methylene Blue as a Diagnostic Aid in the Early Detection and Screening of Oral

Squamous Cell Carcinoma and Precancer Lesions." *Journal of the Chinese Medical Association* 70 (11): 497–503. https://doi.org/10.1016/S1726-4901(08)70048-0.

Chiappin, Silvia, Giorgia Antonelli, Rosalba Gatti, and Elio F. De Palo. 2007. "Saliva Specimen: A New Laboratory Tool for Diagnostic and Basic Investigation." *Clinica Chimica Acta* 383 (1–2): 30–40. https://doi.org/10.1016/j.cca.2007.04.011.

Chien, Ming Hsien, Chung Han Hsin, Lin Shih-Shen Chou, Tsung Te Chung, Chien Huang Lin, Meng Shih Weng, Ming Yung Chou, Mu Kuan Chen, and Shun Fa Yang. 2012. "Interleukin-23 Receptor Polymorphism as a Risk Factor for Oral Cancer Susceptibility." *Head and Neck* 34 (4): 551–56. https://doi.org/10.1002/hed.21779.

Chu, Hao Wei, Kai Ping Chang, Chia Wei Hsu, Ian Yi Feng Chang, Hao Ping Liu, Yi Ting Chen, and Chih Ching Wu. 2019. "Identification of Salivary Biomarkers for Oral Cancer Detection with Untargeted and Targeted Quantitative Proteomics Approaches." *Molecular and Cellular Proteomics* 18 (9): 1796–1806. https://doi.org/10.1074/mcp.RA119.001530.

Cohen, Joshua D., Ammar A. Javed, Christopher Thoburn, Fay Wong, Jeanne Tie, Peter Gibbs, C. Max Schmidt, et al. 2017. "Combined Circulating Tumor DNA and Protein Biomarker-Based Liquid Biopsy for the Earlier Detection of Pancreatic Cancers." *Proceedings of the National Academy of Sciences of the United States of America* 114 (38): 10202–7. https://doi.org/10.1073/pnas.1704961114.

Cristaldi, Marta, Rodolfo Mauceri, Olga Di Fede, Giovanna Giuliana, Giuseppina Campisi, and Vera Panzarella. 2019. "Salivary Biomarkers for Oral Squamous Cell Carcinoma Diagnosis and Follow-up: Current Status and Perspectives." *Frontiers in Psychology* 10. https://doi.org/10.3389/fphys.2019.01476.

Czerninski, R, S Krichevsky, Y Ashhab, D Gazit, V Patel, and D Ben-Yehuda. 2009. "Promoter Hypermethylation of Mismatch Repair Genes, *HMLH1* and *HMSH2* in Oral Squamous Cell Carcinoma." *Oral Diseases* 15 (3): 206–13. https://doi.org/10.1111/j.1601-0825.2008.01510.x.

d'Errico, Margherita, Elizabeth Alwers, Yan Zhang, Dominic Edelmann, Hermann Brenner, and Michael Hoffmeister. 2020. "Identification of Prognostic DNA Methylation Biomarkers in Patients with Gastrointestinal Adenocarcinomas: A Systematic Review of Epigenome-Wide Studies." *Cancer Treatment Reviews*. W.B. Saunders Ltd. https://doi.org/10.1016/j.ctrv.2019.101933.

Datta, Sayantan, Anindita Ray, Richa Singh, Pinaki Mondal, Analabha Basu, Navonil De Sarkar, Mousumi Majumder, et al. 2015. "Sequence and Expression Variations in 23 Genes Involved in Mitochondrial and Non-Mitochondrial Apoptotic Pathways and Risk of Oral Leukoplakia and Cancer." *Mitochondrion* 25: 28–33. https://doi.org/10.1016/j.mito.2015.09.001.

Delavarian, Zahra, Nooshin Mohtasham, Pegah Mosannen-Mozaffari, Atessa Pakfetrat, Mohammad Taghi Shakeri, and Rasoul Ghafoorian-Maddah. 2010. "Evaluation of the Diagnostic Value of a Modified Liquid-Based Cytology Using OralCDx ® Brush in Early Detection of Oral Potentially Malignant Lesions and Oral Cancer." *Medicina Oral, Patologia Oral y Cirugia Bucal* 15 (5). https://doi.org/10.4317/medoral.15.e671.

Dinger, Marcel E., Timothy R. Mercer, and John S. Mattick. 2008. "RNAs as Extracellular Signaling Molecules." *Journal of Molecular Endocrinology* 40 (3–4): 151–59. https://doi.org/10.1677/JME-07-0160.

Dou, Zhichao, Shaoming Li, Wenhao Ren, Qibo Wang, Jiacheng Liu, Xinjuan Kong, Ling Gao, and Keqian Zhi. 2019. "Decreased Expression of Hsa_circ_0072387 as a Valuable Predictor for Oral Squamous Cell Carcinoma." *Oral Diseases* 25 (5): 1302–8. https://doi.org/10.1111/odi.13094.

Du, Ge Fei, Cheng Zhang Li, Han Zheng Chen, Xin Ming Chen, Qun Xiao, Zheng Guo Cao, Shu Huan Shang, and Xia Cai. 2007. "Rose Bengal Staining in Detection of Oral Precancerous and Malignant Lesions with Colorimetric Evaluation: A Pilot Study." *International Journal of Cancer* 120 (9): 1958–63. https://doi.org/10.1002/ijc.22467.

Easton, D. F., D. Ford, D. T. Bishop, N. Haites, B. Milner, L. Allan, D. F. Easton, et al. 1995. "Breast and Ovarian Cancer Incidence in BRCA1-Mutation Carriers." *American Journal of Human Genetics* 56 (1): 265–71.

El-Khoury, Victoria, Anna Schritz, Sang Yoon Kim, Antoine Lesur, Katriina Sertamo, François Bernardin, Konstantinos Petritis, et al. 2020. "Identification of a Blood-Based Protein Biomarker Panel for Lung Cancer Detection." *Cancers* 12 (6): 1–15. https://doi.org/10.3390/cancers12061629.

Elashoff, David, Uttam Sinha, David T W Wong, Yang Li, Myungshin Oh, Maie AR St John, Xiaofeng Zhou, Elliot Abemayor, and David T Wong. 2006. "Serum Circulating Human MRNA Profiling and Its Utility for Oral Cancer Detection." *Article in Journal of Clinical Oncology* 24: 1754–60. https://doi.org/10.1200/JCO.2005.03.7598.

Ellinger, Jörg, Philip Kahl, Johannes Von Der Gathen, Sebastian Rogenhofer, Lukas C. Heukamp, Ines Gütgemann, Bernhard Walter, et al. 2010. "Global Levels of Histone Modifications Predict Prostate Cancer Recurrence." *Prostate* 70 (1): 61–69. https://doi.org/10.1002/pros.21038.

Elsheikh, Somaia E., Andrew R. Green, Emad A. Rakha, Des G. Powe, Rabab A. Ahmed, Hilary M. Collins, Daniele Soria, et al. 2009. "Global Histone Modifications in Breast Cancer Correlate with Tumor Phenotypes, Prognostic Factors, and Patient Outcome." *Cancer Research* 69 (9): 3802–9. https://doi.org/10.1158/0008-5472.CAN-08-3907.

Epstein, Joel B., Robert V. Kish, Lucy Hallajian, and James Sciubba. 2015. "Head and Neck, Oral, and Oropharyngeal Cancer: A Review of Medicolegal Cases." *Oral Surgery, Oral Medicine, Oral Pathology and Oral Radiology* 119 (2): 177–86. https://doi.org/10.1016/j.oooo.2014.10.002.

Epstein, Joel B., Crispian Scully, and John Spinelli. 1992. "Toluidine Blue and Lugol's Iodine Application in the Assessment of Oral Malignant Disease and Lesions at Risk of Malignancy." *Journal of Oral Pathology*

& *Medicine* 21 (4): 160–63. https://doi.org/10.1111/j.1600-0714.1992.tb00094.x.

Fang, Zhengyu, Lamei Wu, Luo Wang, Yang Yang, Yusheng Meng, and Hongyu Yang. 2014. “Increased Expression of the Long Non-Coding RNA UCA1 in Tongue Squamous Cell Carcinomas: A Possible Correlation with Cancer Metastasis.” *Oral Surgery, Oral Medicine, Oral Pathology and Oral Radiology* 117 (1): 89–95. https://doi.org/10.1016/j.oooo.2013.09.007.

Farooq, Imran, and Amr Bugshan. 2020. “Oral Squamous Cell Carcinoma: Metastasis, Potentially Associated Malignant Disorders, Etiology and Recent Advancements in Diagnosis.” *F1000Research* 9. https://doi.org/10.12688/f1000research.22941.1.

Fine, Jo David, Lorraine B. Johnson, Madeline Weiner, Kuo Ping Li, and Chirayath Suchindran. 2009. “Epidermolysis Bullosa and the Risk of Life-Threatening Cancers: The National EB Registry Experience, 1986-2006.” *Journal of the American Academy of Dermatology* 60 (2): 203–11. https://doi.org/10.1016/j.jaad.2008.09.035.

Fitzpatrick, Sarah G., Stanley A. Hirsch, and Sara C. Gordon. 2014. “The Malignant Transformation of Oral Lichen Planus and Oral Lichenoid Lesions A Systematic Review.” *Journal of the American Dental Association* 145 (1): 45–56. https://doi.org/10.14219/jada.2013.10.

Flynn, Ryan A., and Howard Y. Chang. 2014. “Long Noncoding RNAs in Cell-Fate Programming and Reprogramming.” *Cell Stem Cell.* Cell Press. https://doi.org/10.1016/j.stem.2014.05.014.

Fontes, Karla Bianca Fernandes da Costa, Karin Soares Gonçalves Cunha, Fabiana Resende Rodrigues, Licínio Esmeraldo da Silva, and Eliane Pedra Dias. 2013. “Concordance between Cytopathology and Incisional Biopsy in the Diagnosis of Oral Squamous Cell Carcinoma.” *Brazilian Oral Research* 27 (2): 122–27. https://doi.org/10.1590/S1806-83242013000100018.

Foster, Jared C., Jeremy M.G. Taylor, and Stephen J. Ruberg. 2011. “Subgroup Identification from Randomized Clinical Trial Data.” *Statistics in Medicine* 30 (24): 2867–80. https://doi.org/10.1002/sim.4322.

Fu, Liyun, Ting Yao, Qingqing Chen, Xiaoyan Mo, Yaoren Hu, and Junming Guo. 2017. "Screening Differential Circular RNA Expression Profiles Reveals Hsa_circ_0004018 Is Associated with Hepatocellular Carcinoma." *Oncotarget* 8 (35): 58405–16. https://doi.org/10.18632/oncotarget.16881.

Fu, Ting Ying, I. Chien Hsieh, Jiin Tsuey Cheng, Meng Han Tsai, Yu Yi Hou, Jang Hwa Lee, Huei Han Liou, et al. 2016. "Association of OCT4, SOX2, and NANOG Expression with Oral Squamous Cell Carcinoma Progression." *Journal of Oral Pathology and Medicine* 45 (2): 89–95. https://doi.org/10.1111/jop.12335.

Fuchs, Aaron, and Ellen Marmur. 2007. "The Kinetics of Skin Cancer: Progression of Actinic Keratosis to Squamous Cell Carcinoma." *Dermatologic Surgery* 33 (9): 1099–1101. https://doi.org/10.1111/j.1524-4725.2007.33224.x.

Gainor, Justin F., Dan L. Longo, and Bruce A. Chabner. 2014. "Pharmacodynamic Biomarkers: Falling Short of the Mark?" *Clinical Cancer Research* 20 (10): 2587–94. https://doi.org/10.1158/1078-0432.CCR-13-3132.

Gao, Ling, Wenhao Ren, Su'e Chang, Bo Guo, Shuo Huang, Menghe Li, Youmin Guo, et al. 2013. "Downregulation of MiR-145 Expression in Oral Squamous Cell Carcinomas and Its Clinical Significance." *Onkologie* 36 (4): 194–99. https://doi.org/10.1159/000349956.

Gaur, P., M. Mittal, B. K. Mohanti, and Satya N. Das. 2011. "Functional Variants of IL4 and IL6 Genes and Risk of Tobacco-Related Oral Carcinoma in High-Risk Asian Indians." *Oral Diseases* 17 (7): 720–26. https://doi.org/10.1111/j.1601-0825.2011.01831.x.

Gayther, Simon A, Honglin Song, Susan J Ramus, Susan Krüger Kjaer, Alice S Whittemore, Lydia Quaye, Jonathan Tyrer, et al. 2007. *Tagging Single Nucleotide Polymorphisms in Cell Cycle Control Genes and Susceptibility to Invasive Epithelial Ovarian Cancer.* https://doi.org/10.1158/0008-5472.CAN-06-3261.

Ge, Xiaosong, Yuanbin Chen, Xiaoyu Liao, Deqing Liu, Fangfang Li, Honglian, Ruan, and Weihua Jia. 2013. "Overexpression of Long Noncoding RNA PCAT-1 Is a Novel Biomarker of Poor Prognosis in

Patients with Colorectal Cancer." *Springer* 30 (2): 588. https://doi.org/10.1007/s12032-013-0588-6.

Ghaffari, Maryam, Milad Asadi, Dariush Shanehbandi, Soghra Bornehdeli, Mahsa Sadeghzadeh, Haniye Mohammad Reza Khani, and Shahram Ghasembaglou. 2020. "Aberrant Expression of MiR-103, MiR-184, MiR-378, MiR-497 and MiR-506 in Tumor Tissue from Patients with Oral Squamous Cell Carcinoma Regulates the Clinical Picture of the Patients." *Asian Pacific Journal of Cancer Prevention* 21 (5): 1311–15. https://doi.org/10.31557/APJCP.2020.21.5.1311.

González-Ramírez, I., V. Ramírez-Amador, M. E. Irigoyen-Camacho, Y. Sánchez-Pérez, G. Anaya-Saavedra, M. Granados-García, F. García-Vázquez, and C. M. García-Cuellar. 2011. "HMLH1 Promoter Methylation Is an Early Event in Oral Cancer." *Oral Oncology* 47 (1): 22–26. https://doi.org/10.1016/j.oraloncology.2010.10.002.

Goodson, M. L., and P. J. Thomson. 2011. "Management of Oral Carcinoma: Benefits of Early Precancerous Intervention." *British Journal of Oral and Maxillofacial Surgery* 49 (2): 88–91. https://doi.org/10.1016/j.bjoms.2009.12.014.

Goossens, Nicolas, Shigeki Nakagawa, Xiaochen Sun, and Yujin Hoshida. 2015. "Cancer Biomarker Discovery and Validation." *Translational Cancer Research* 4 (3): 256–69. https://doi.org/10.3978/j.issn.2218-676X.2015.06.04.

Grajewski, S., and D. Groneberg. 2009. "Leukoplakia and Erythroplakia Two Orale Precursor Lesions [Leukoplakie Und Erythroplakie Zwei Orale Räkursorläsionen]." *Laryngo- Rhino- Otologie* 88 (10): 666–75. http://www.scopus.com/inward/record.url?eid=2-s2.0-70449380821&partnerID=40&md5=c4345587e183c639cb6059fbb1630f28.

Grochola, Lukasz F., Jorge Zeron-Medina, Sophie Mériaux, and Gareth L. Bond. 2010. "Single-Nucleotide Polymorphisms in the P53 Signaling Pathway." *Cold Spring Harbor Perspectives in Biology*. https://doi.org/10.1101/cshperspect.a001032.

Guo, Theresa, Daria A. Gaykalova, Michael Considine, Sarah Wheelan, Aparna Pallavajjala, Justin A. Bishop, William H. Westra, et al. 2016. "Characterization of Functionally Active Gene Fusions in Human

Papillomavirus Related Oropharyngeal Squamous Cell Carcinoma." *International Journal of Cancer* 139 (2): 373–82. https://doi.org/10.1002/ijc.30081.

Gupta, P. C., F. S. Mehta, and D. K. Daftary. 1980. "Incidence Rates of Oral Cancer and Natural History of Oral Precancerous Lesions in a 10-Year Follow-up Study of Indian Villagers." *Community Dentistry and Oral Epidemiology* 8 (6): 287–333. https://doi.org/10.1111/j.1600-0528.1980.tb01302.x.

Hadzic, Sanja, Mirjana GojkovVukelic, Enes Pasic, and Almir Dervisevic. 2017. "Importance of Early Detection of Potentially Malignant Lesions in the Prevention of Oral Cancer." *Materia Socio Medica* 29 (2): 129. https://doi.org/10.5455/msm.2017.29.129-133.

Haldrup, Christa, Anne L. Pedersen, Nadia Øgaard, Siri H. Strand, Søren Høyer, Michael Borre, Torben F. Ørntoft, and Karina D. Sørensen. 2018. "Biomarker Potential of *ST6GALNAC3* and *ZNF660* Promoter Hypermethylation in Prostate Cancer Tissue and Liquid Biopsies." *Molecular Oncology* 12 (4): 545–60. https://doi.org/10.1002/1878-0261.12183.

Hamam, Rimi, Dana Hamam, Khalid A. Alsaleh, Moustapha Kassem, Waleed Zaher, Musaad Alfayez, Abdullah Aldahmash, and Nehad M. Alajez. 2017. "Circulating MicroRNAs in Breast Cancer: Novel Diagnostic and Prognostic Biomarkers." *Cell Death & Disease*. Nature Publishing Group. https://doi.org/10.1038/cddis.2017.440.

Handschel, Jörg, Döne Öz, Natalia Pomjanski, Rita Depprich, Michelle A. Ommerborn, Stefan Braunstein, Norbert R. Kübler, Ulrich Meyer, and Alfred Böcking. 2007. "Additional Use of DNA-Image Cytometry Improves the Assessment of Resection Margins." *Journal of Oral Pathology and Medicine* 36 (8): 472–75. https://doi.org/10.1111/j.1600-0714.2007.00564.x.

Hanken, Henning, Juliane Kraatz, Ralf Smeets, Max Heiland, Marco Blessmann, Wolfgang Eichhorn, Till S. Clauditz, Alexander Gröbe, Andreas Kolk, and Madiha Rana. 2013. "The Detection of Oral Pre-Malignant Lesions with an Autofluorescence Based Imaging System

(VELscopeTM) - a Single Blinded Clinical Evaluation." *Head and Face Medicine* 9 (1). https://doi.org/10.1186/1746-160X-9-23.

Happle, R. 1999. "Loss of Heterozygosity in Human Skin." *Journal of the American Academy of Dermatology* 41 (2 I): 143–61. https://doi.org/10.1016/S0190-9622(99)70042-3.

Harishankar, M. K., A. Mathan Mohan, A. Vinod Krishnan, and Arikketh Devi. 2019. "Downregulation of Notch4 – a Prognostic Marker in Distinguishing Oral Verrucous Carcinoma from Oral Squamous Cell Carcinoma." *Brazilian Journal of Otorhinolaryngology*. https://doi.org/10.1016/j.bjorl.2017.09.005.

He, Lihong, Fan Ping, Zhaona Fan, Chi Zhang, Miao Deng, Bin Cheng, and Juan Xia. 2020. "Salivary Exosomal MiR-24-3p Serves as a Potential Detective Biomarker for Oral Squamous Cell Carcinoma Screening." *Biomedicine and Pharmacotherapy* 121 (January): 109553. https://doi.org/10.1016/j.biopha.2019.109553.

Henry, N. Lynn, and Daniel F. Hayes. 2012. "Cancer Biomarkers." *Molecular Oncology* 6 (2): 140–46. https://doi.org/10.1016/j.molonc.2012.01.010.

Hsu, Han Jen, Yi Hsin Yang, Tien Yu Shieh, Chung Ho Chen, Yu Hsun Kao, Chia Fu Yang, and Edward Cheng Chuan Ko. 2015. "TGF-B1 and IL-10 Single Nucleotide Polymorphisms as Risk Factors for Oral Cancer in Taiwanese." *Kaohsiung Journal of Medical Sciences* 31 (3): 123–29. https://doi.org/10.1016/j.kjms.2014.12.003.

Hu, Chengping, Silke Meiners, Christina Lukas, Georgios T. Stathopoulos, and Jie Chen. 2020. "Role of Exosomal MicroRNAs in Lung Cancer Biology and Clinical Applications." *Cell Proliferation* 53 (6): e12828. https://doi.org/10.1111/cpr.12828.

Hu, Shen, Martha Arellano, Pinmanee Boontheung, Jianghua Wang, Hui Zhou, Jiang Jiang, David Elashoff, Roger Wei, Joseph A. Loo, and David T. Wong. 2008. "Salivary Proteomics for Oral Cancer Biomarker Discovery." *Clinical Cancer Research* 14 (19): 6246–52. https://doi.org/10.1158/1078-0432.CCR-07-5037.

Hu, Wenqian, Juan R Alvarez-Dominguez, and Harvey F Lodish. 2012. "Regulation of Mammalian Cell Differentiation by Long Non-coding

RNAs." *EMBO Reports* 13 (11): 971–83. https://doi.org/10.1038/embor.2012.145.

Huang, Guang Zhao, Qing Qing Wu, Ze Nan Zheng, Ting Ru Shao, and Xiao Zhi Lv. 2019. "Identification of Candidate Biomarkers and Analysis of Prognostic Values in Oral Squamous Cell Carcinoma." *Frontiers in Oncology* 9 (OCT). https://doi.org/10.3389/fonc.2019.01054.

Huang, Shi wei, Ni da Ali, Lily Zhong, and Jian Shi. 2018. "MicroRNAs as Biomarkers for Human Glioblastoma: Progress and Potential." *Acta Pharmacologica Sinica* 39 (9): 1405–13. https://doi.org/10.1038/aps.2017.173.

Huang, Shiang Fu, Fu Chan Wei, Chun Ta Liao, Hung Ming Wang, Chien Yu Lin, Steven Lo, Jung Ju Huang, et al. 2012. "Risk Stratification in Oral Cavity Squamous Cell Carcinoma by Preoperative CRP and SCC Antigen Levels." *Annals of Surgical Oncology* 19 (12): 3856–64. https://doi.org/10.1245/s10434-012-2392-5.

Hunter, Keith D., E. Ken Parkinson, and Paul R. Harrison. 2005. "Profiling Early Head and Neck Cancer." *Nature Reviews Cancer* 5 (2): 127–35. https://doi.org/10.1038/nrc1549.

Jackson, Robert C. 2012. "Pharmacodynamic Modelling of Biomarker Data in Oncology." *ISRN Pharmacology* 2012: 1–12. https://doi.org/10.5402/2012/590626.

Janssen, A., and R. H. Medema. 2013. "Genetic Instability: Tipping the Balance." *Oncogene* 32 (38): 4459–70. https://doi.org/10.1038/onc.2012.576.

Jayaprakash, Chinchu, Raghu Radhakrishnan, Satadru Ray, and Kapaettu Satyamoorthy. 2017. "Promoter Methylation of MGMT in Oral Carcinoma: A Population-Based Study and Meta-Analysis." *Archives of Oral Biology* 80 (August): 197–208. https://doi.org/10.1016/j.archoralbio.2017.04.006.

Jerjes, Waseem, Tahwinder Upile, Aviva Petrie, Andrew Riskalla, Zaid Hamdoon, Michael Vourvachis, Kostas Karavidas, et al. 2010. "Clinicopathological Parameters, Recurrence, Locoregional and Distant

Metastasis in 115 T1-T2 Oral Squamous Cell Carcinoma Patients." *Head and Neck Oncology* 2 (1). https://doi.org/10.1186/1758-3284-2-9.

Jessner, Wolfgang, Harald Vogelsang, Andreas Püspök, Peter Ferenci, Alfred Gangl, Gottfried Novacek, Astrid Bodisch, and Etienne Wenzl. 2003. "Plummer-Vinson Syndrome Associated with Celiac Disease and Complicated by Postcricoid Carcinoma and Carcinoma of the Tongue [7]." *American Journal of Gastroenterology* 98 (5): 1208–9. https://doi.org/10.1111/j.1572-0241.2003.07438.x.

Jha, Ritu, Poonam Gaur, Suresh Chandra Sharma, and Satya Narayan Das. 2013. "Single Nucleotide Polymorphism in HMLH1 Promoter and Risk of Tobacco-Related Oral Carcinoma in High-Risk Asian Indians." *Gene* 526 (2): 223–27. https://doi.org/10.1016/j.gene.2013.05.014.

Jiang, Tao, Guoxia Liu, Lin Wang, and Hongchen Liu. 2015. "Elevated Serum Gas 6 Is a Novel Prognostic Biomarker in Patients with Oral Squamous Cell Carcinoma." *PLoS ONE* 10 (7). https://doi.org/10.1371/journal.pone.0133940.

John, Maie A.R. St., Yang Li, Xiaofeng Zhou, Paul Denny, Chih Ming Ho, Carlo Montemagno, Wenyuan Shi, et al. 2004. "Interleukin 6 and Interleukin 8 as Potential Biomarkers for Oral Cavity and Oropharyngeal Squamous Cell Carcinoma." *Archives of Otolaryngology - Head and Neck Surgery* 130 (8): 929–35. https://doi.org/10.1001/archotol.130.8.929.

Juźwik, Camille A., Sienna S. Drake, Yang Zhang, Nicolas Paradis-Isler, Alexandra Sylvester, Alexandre Amar-Zifkin, Chelsea Douglas, Barbara Morquette, Craig S. Moore, and Alyson E. Fournier. 2019. "MicroRNA Dysregulation in Neurodegenerative Diseases: A Systematic Review." *Progress in Neurobiology*. Elsevier Ltd. https://doi.org/10.1016/j.pneurobio.2019.101664.

Kadhim Al-Malkey, Maysaa, Ahmed AH Abbas, Noorulhuda F Khalaf, Istabraq AH Mubarak, and Iftikhar AH Jasim. 2015. "Expression Analysis of Salivary Microrna-31 in Oral Cancer Patients." *Int. J. Curr. Microbiol. App. Sci*. Vol. 4.

Kamel HF, Al-Amodi HS. n.d. Cancer Biomarkers. In *Role of Biomarkers in Medicine*. https://doi.org/10.5772/62421.

Karimi, Abbas, Naghmeh Bahrami, Amirsalar Sayedyahossein, and Samira Derakhshan. 2020. "Evaluation of Circulating Serum 3 Types of MicroRNA as Biomarkers of Oral Squamous Cell Carcinoma; A Pilot Study." *Journal of Oral Pathology and Medicine* 49 (1): 43–48. https://doi.org/10.1111/jop.12959.

Karimi, Shirin, Abdolreza Mohamadnia, Seyed Alireza Nadji, Reza Yadegarazari, Adnan Khosravi, Naghmeh Bahrami, and Massoud Saidijam. 2015. "Expression of Two Basic MRNA Biomarkers in Peripheral Blood of Patients with Non-Small Cell Lung Cancer Detected by Real-Time RT-PCR, Individually and Simultaneously." *Iranian Biomedical Journal* 19 (1): 17–22. https://doi.org/10.6091/ibj.1397.2014.

Kashyap, Dharambir, and Harmandeep Kaur. 2020. "Cell-Free MiRNAs as Non-Invasive Biomarkers in Breast Cancer: Significance in Early Diagnosis and Metastasis Prediction." *Life Sciences*. Elsevier Inc. https://doi.org/10.1016/j.lfs.2020.117417.

Kawahara, Rebeca, James G. Bollinger, César Rivera, Ana Carolina P. Ribeiro, Thaís Bianca Brandão, Adriana F.Paes Leme, and Michael J. Maccoss. 2016. "A Targeted Proteomic Strategy for the Measurement of Oral Cancer Candidate Biomarkers in Human Saliva." *Proteomics* 16 (1): 159–73. https://doi.org/10.1002/pmic.201500224.

Kayahara, H., H. Yamagata, H. Tanioka, T. Miki, and H. Hamakawa. 2001. "Frequent Loss of Heterozygosity at 3p25-P26 Is Associated with Invasive Oral Squamous Cell Carcinoma." *Journal of Human Genetics* 46 (6): 335–41. https://doi.org/10.1007/s100380170069.

Kerr, Ar, S. Warnakulasuriya, Aj Mighell, T. Dietrich, M. Nasser, J. Rimal, A. Jalil, et al. 2011. "A Systematic Review of Medical Interventions for Oral Submucous Fibrosis and Future Research Opportunities." *Oral Diseases* 17 (SUPPL. 1): 42–57. https://doi.org/10.1111/j.1601-0825.2011.01791.x.

Kietthubthew, Suparp, Hutcha Sriplung, William W. Au, and Takafumi Ishida. 2006. "Polymorphism in DNA Repair Genes and Oral Squamous Cell Carcinoma in Thailand." *International Journal of Hygiene and*

Environmental Health 209 (1): 21–29. https://doi.org/10.1016/j.ijheh.2005.06.002.

Kim, Jo Heon, Min Ho Shin, Sun Seog Kweon, Min Ho Park, Jung Han Yoon, Ji Shin Lee, Chan Choi, Mary Jo Fackler, and Saraswati Sukumar. 2010. "Evaluation of Promoter Hypermethylation Detection in Serum as a Diagnostic Tool for Breast Carcinoma in Korean Women." *Gynecologic Oncology* 118 (2): 176–81. https://doi.org/10.1016/j.ygyno.2010.04.016.

Kloten, Vera, Birte Becker, Kirsten Winner, Michael G. Schrauder, Peter A. Fasching, Tobias Anzeneder, Jürgen Veeck, Arndt Hartmann, Ruth Knüchel, and Edgar Dahl. 2013. "Promoter Hypermethylation of the Tumor-Suppressor Genes ITIH5, DKK3, and RASSF1A as Novel Biomarkers for Blood-Based Breast Cancer Screening." *Breast Cancer Research* 15 (1): 1–11. https://doi.org/10.1186/bcr3375.

Koivunen, Jussi P., Craig Mermel, Kreshnik Zejnullahu, Carly Murphy, Eugene Lifshits, Alison J. Holmes, Hwan Geun Choi, et al. 2008. "EML4-ALK Fusion Gene and Efficacy of an ALK Kinase Inhibitor in Lung Cancer." *Clinical Cancer Research* 14 (13): 4275–83. https://doi.org/10.1158/1078-0432.CCR-08-0168.

Lai, Chih Ho, Nai Wen Chang, Chin Fen Lin, Chia Der Lin, Ying Ju Lin, Lei Wan, Jim Jinn Chyuan Sheu, et al. 2010. "Proteomics-Based Identification of Haptoglobin as a Novel Plasma Biomarker in Oral Squamous Cell Carcinoma." *Clinica Chimica Acta* 411 (13–14): 984–91. https://doi.org/10.1016/j.cca.2010.03.028.

Lajer, C. B., F. C. Nielsen, L. Friis-Hansen, B. Norrild, R. Borup, E. Garnæs, M. Rossing, et al. 2011. "Different MiRNA Signatures of Oral and Pharyngeal Squamous Cell Carcinomas: A Prospective Translational Study." *British Journal of Cancer* 104 (5): 830–40. https://doi.org/10.1038/bjc.2011.29.

Lauritano, D., A. Lucchese, M. Contaldo, R. Serpico, L. L.O. Muzio, F. Biolcati, and F. Carinci. 2016. "Moral Squamous Cell Carcinoma: Diagnostic Markers and Prognostic Indicators." *Journal of Biological Regulators and Homeostatic Agents* 30 (2): 169–76.

Le, Han Bo, Wang Yu Zhu, Dong Dong Chen, Jian Ying He, Yan Yan Huang, Xiao Guang Liu, and Yong Kui Zhang. 2012. "Evaluation of Dynamic Change of Serum MiR-21 and MiR-24 in Pre- and Post-Operative Lung Carcinoma Patients." *Medical Oncology* 29 (5): 3190–97. https://doi.org/10.1007/s12032-012-0303-z.

Lengauer, Christoph, Kenneth W. Kinzler, and Bert Vogelstein. 1998. "Genetic Instabilities in Human Cancers." *Nature* 396 (6712): 643–49. https://doi.org/10.1038/25292.

Lewis, Benjamin P., I. Hung Shih, Matthew W. Jones-Rhoades, David P. Bartel, and Christopher B. Burge. 2003. "Prediction of Mammalian MicroRNA Targets." *Cell* 115 (7): 787–98. https://doi.org/10.1016/S0092-8674(03)01018-3.

Li, Bowen, Feng Wang, Xiang Li, Shuai Sun, Yuehong Shen, and Hongyu Yang. 2018. "Hsa_circ_0008309 May Be a Potential Biomarker for Oral Squamous Cell Carcinoma." *Disease Markers* 2018. https://doi.org/10.1155/2018/7496890.

Li, Chunmei, Ya Zheng, Ke Pu, Da Zhao, Yuping Wang, Quanlin Guan, and Yongning Zhou. 2020. "A Four-DNA Methylation Signature as a Novel Prognostic Biomarker for Survival of Patients with Gastric Cancer." *Cancer Cell International* 20 (1): 88. https://doi.org/10.1186/s12935-020-1156-8.

Li, Gang, Hao Shi, Xinyi Wang, Bei Wang, Qianqian Qu, Haiyang Geng, and Hongjun Sun. 2019. "Identification of Diagnostic Long Non-coding RNA Biomarkers in Patients with Hepatocellular Carcinoma." *Molecular Medicine Reports* 20 (2): 1121–30. https://doi.org/10.3892/mmr.2019.10307.

Li, Lin, and Zhong Ti Zhang. 2020. "Hsa_circ_0086414 Might Be a Diagnostic Biomarker of Oral Squamous Cell Carcinoma." *Medical Science Monitor* 26 (January). https://doi.org/10.12659/MSM.919383.

Li, Ning, Chao Zhang, Zhaoquan Chen, Lilu Bai, Min Nie, Bin Zhou, and Huanxi Xu. 2015. "Interleukin 17A and Interleukin 17F Polymorphisms Are Associated with Oral Squamous Cell Carcinoma Susceptibility in a Chinese Population." *Journal of Oral and Maxillofacial Surgery* 73 (2): 267–73. https://doi.org/10.1016/j.joms.2014.09.009.

Li, Peifei, Shengcan Chen, Huilin Chen, Xiaoyan Mo, Tianwen Li, Yongfu Shao, Bingxiu Xiao, and Junming Guo. 2015. "Using Circular RNA as a Novel Type of Biomarker in the Screening of Gastric Cancer." *Clinica Chimica Acta* 444 (April): 132–36. https://doi.org/10.1016/j.cca.2015.02.018.

Li, Xiaohong, Patricia L. Blount, Thomas L. Vaughan, and Brian J. Reid. 2011. "Application of Biomarkers in Cancer Risk Management: Evaluation from Stochastic Clonal Evolutionary and Dynamic System Optimization Points of View." *PLoS Computational Biology* 7 (2). https://doi.org/10.1371/journal.pcbi.1001087.

Li, Yue, Xiaofang Cao, and Hao Li. 2020. "Identification and Validation of Novel Long Non-Coding RNA Biomarkers for Early Diagnosis of Oral Squamous Cell Carcinoma." *Frontiers in Bioengineering and Biotechnology* 8 (April). https://doi.org/10.3389/fbioe.2020.00256.

Lin, Jie, Dongping Cai, Wei Li, Ting Yu, Hui Mao, Shan Jiang, and Bin Xiao. 2019. "Plasma Circular RNA Panel Acts as a Novel Diagnostic Biomarker for Colorectal Cancer." *Clinical Biochemistry* 74 (December): 60–68. https://doi.org/10.1016/j.clinbiochem.2019.10.012.

Lin, Jin Ching, Chen Chi Wang, Rong San Jiang, Wen Yi Wang, and Shih An Liu. 2016. "Microsatellite Alteration in Head and Neck Squamous Cell Carcinoma Patients from a Betel Quid-Prevalent Region." *Scientific Reports* 6. https://doi.org/10.1038/srep22614.

Lin, Kenneth, Robert Lipsitz, Therese Miller, and Supriya Janakiraman. 2008. "Benefits and Harms of Prostate-Specific Antigen Screening for Prostate Cancer: An Evidence Update for the U.S. Preventive Services Task Force." *Annals of Internal Medicine* 149 (3): 192–99. https://doi.org/10.7326/0003-4819-149-3-200808050-00009.

Lin, Shu Chun, Chung Ji Liu, Jung An Lin, Wei Fan Chiang, Pei Shih Hung, and Kuo Wei Chang. 2010. "MiR-24 up-Regulation in Oral Carcinoma: Positive Association from Clinical and in Vitro Analysis." *Oral Oncology* 46 (3): 204–8. https://doi.org/10.1016/j.oraloncology.2009.12.005.

Lingen, Mark W., John R. Kalmar, Theodore Karrison, and Paul M. Speight. 2008. "Critical Evaluation of Diagnostic Aids for the Detection of Oral Cancer." *Oral Oncology* 44 (1): 10–22. https://doi.org/10.1016/j.oraloncology.2007.06.011.

Lingen, Mw, A. Pinto, Ra Mendes, R. Franchini, R. Czerninski, Wm Tilakaratne, M. Partridge, De Peterson, and S. B. Woo. 2011. "Genetics/Epigenetics of Oral Premalignancy: Current Status and Future Research." *Oral Diseases* 17 (SUPPL. 1): 7–22. https://doi.org/10.1111/j.1601-0825.2011.01789.x.

Lipkovich, Ilya, Alex Dmitrienko, Jonathan Denne, and Gregory Enas. 2011. "Subgroup Identification Based on Differential Effect Search-A Recursive Partitioning Method for Establishing Response to Treatment in Patient Subpopulations." *Statistics in Medicine* 30 (21): 2601–21. https://doi.org/10.1002/sim.4289.

Liu, Bin, Chun Feng Pan, Zhi Cheng He, Jun Wang, Peng Li Wang, Teng Ma, Yang Xia, and Yi Jiang Chen. 2016. "Long Noncoding RNA-LET Suppresses Tumor Growth and EMT in Lung Adenocarcinoma." *BioMed Research International* 2016. https://doi.org/10.1155/2016/4693471.

Liu, C. J., S. Y. Kao, H. F. Tu, M. M. Tsai, K. W. Chang, and S. C. Lin. 2010. "Increase of MicroRNA MiR-31 Level in Plasma Could Be a Potential Marker of Oral Cancer." *Oral Diseases* 16 (4): 360–64. https://doi.org/10.1111/j.1601-0825.2009.01646.x.

Liu, Chung Ji, Shu Chun Lin, Cheng Chieh Yang, Hui Wen Cheng, and Kuo Wei Chang. 2012. "Exploiting Salivary MiR-31 as a Clinical Biomarker of Oral Squamous Cell Carcinoma." *Head and Neck* 34 (2): 219–24. https://doi.org/10.1002/hed.21713.

Liu, Hanshao, Deji Ye, Aijun Chen, Dan Tan, Wenpeng Zhang, Wenxia Jiang, Mingliang Wang, and Xiaoren Zhang. 2019. "A Pilot Study of New Promising Non-Coding RNA Diagnostic Biomarkers for Early-Stage Colorectal Cancers." *Clinical Chemistry and Laboratory Medicine* 57 (7): 1073–83. https://doi.org/10.1515/cclm-2019-0052.

Liu, Jingwei, Caiyun He, Chengzhong Xing, and Yuan Yuan. 2014. "Nucleotide Excision Repair Related Gene Polymorphisms and Genetic

Susceptibility, Chemotherapeutic Sensitivity and Prognosis of Gastric Cancer." *Mutation Research - Fundamental and Molecular Mechanisms of Mutagenesis*. Elsevier. https://doi.org/10.1016/j.mrfmmm.2014.04.008.

Liu, Yang, Zeng Tong Zhou, Qing Bo He, and Wei Wen Jiang. 2012. "DAPK Promoter Hypermethylation in Tissues and Body Fluids of Oral Precancer Patients." *Medical Oncology* 29 (2): 729–33. https://doi.org/10.1007/s12032-011-9953-5.

Ma, Rui Min, Fan Yang, Du Ping Huang, Min Zheng, and Yi Luan Wang. 2019. "The Prognostic Value of the Expression of SMC4 MRNA in Breast Cancer." *Disease Markers* 2019. https://doi.org/10.1155/2019/2183057.

Macpherson, Lorna M.D. 2018. "Raising Awareness of Oral Cancer from a Public and Health Professional Perspective." *British Dental Journal* 225 (9): 809–14. https://doi.org/10.1038/sj.bdj.2018.919.

Mahmood, Nosheen, Muhammad Hanif, Akhtar Ahmed, Qamar Jamal, Shamim Mushtaq, Adnan Khan, and Muhammad Saqib. 2019. "Circulating MiR-21 as a Prognostic and Predictive Biomarker in Oral Squamous Cell Carcinoma." *Pakistan Journal of Medical Sciences* 35 (5): 1408–12. https://doi.org/10.12669/pjms.35.5.331.

Martin, Christa Lese, Shalini C. Reshmi, Thomas Ried, William Gottberg, John W. Wilson, Jaya K. Reddy, Poornima Khanna, Jonas T. Johnson, Eugene N. Myers, and Susanne M. Gollin. 2008. "Chromosomal Imbalances in Oral Squamous Cell Carcinoma: Examination of 31 Cell Lines and Review of the Literature." *Oral Oncology* 44 (4): 369–82. https://doi.org/10.1016/j.oraloncology.2007.05.003.

Márton, Ildikó Judit, József Horváth, Péter Lábiscsák, Bernadett Márkus, Balázs Dezső, Adrienn Szabó, Ildikó Tar, et al. 2019. "Salivary IL-6 MRNA Is a Robust Biomarker in Oral Squamous Cell Carcinoma." *Journal of Clinical Medicine* 8 (11): 1958. https://doi.org/10.3390/jcm8111958.

Maruvada, Padma, Wendy Wang, Paul D. Wagner, and Sudhir Srivastava. 2005. "Biomarkers in Molecular Medicine: Cancer Detection and

Diagnosis." *BioTechniques* 38 (4S): S9–15. https://doi.org/10.2144/05384SU04.

Mashberg, Arthur. 1981. "Tolonium (Toluidine Blue) Rinse—A Screening Method for Recognition of Squamous Carcinoma: Continuing Study of Oral Cancer IV." *JAMA: The Journal of the American Medical Association* 245 (23): 2408–10. https://doi.org/10.1001/jama.1981.03310480024019.

Mawardi, H., S. Elad, M. E. Correa, K. Stevenson, S. B. Woo, S. Almazrooa, R. Haddad, J. H. Antin, R. Soiffer, and N. Treister. 2011. "Oral Epithelial Dysplasia and Squamous Cell Carcinoma Following Allogeneic Hematopoietic Stem Cell Transplantation: Clinical Presentation and Treatment Outcomes." *Bone Marrow Transplantation* 46 (6): 884–91. https://doi.org/10.1038/bmt.2011.77.

Meij, E. H. van der, H. Mast, and I. van der Waal. 2007. "The Possible Premalignant Character of Oral Lichen Planus and Oral Lichenoid Lesions: A Prospective Five-Year Follow-up Study of 192 Patients." *Oral Oncology* 43 (8): 742–48. https://doi.org/10.1016/j.oraloncology.2006.09.006.

MILLARD, L. G., and D. J. BARKER. 1978. "Development of Squamous Cell Carcinoma in Chronic Discoid Lupus Erythematosus." *Clinical and Experimental Dermatology* 3 (2): 161–66. https://doi.org/10.1111/j.1365-2230.1978.tb01480.x.

Mishra, Amrendra, Harshini Sriram, Pinal Chandarana, Vivek Tanavde, Rekha V. Kumar, Ashok Gopinath, Raman Govindarajan, S. Ramaswamy, and Subhashini Sadasivam. 2018. "Decreased Expression of Cell Adhesion Genes in Cancer Stem-like Cells Isolated from Primary Oral Squamous Cell Carcinomas." *Tumor Biology* 40 (6). https://doi.org/10.1177/1010428318780859.

Misonou, Yoshiko, Kyoko Shida, Hiroaki Korekane, Yosuke Seki, Shingo Noura, Masayuki Ohue, and Yasuhide Miyamoto. 2009. "Comprehensive Clinico-Glycomic Study of 16 Colorectal Cancer Specimens: Elucidation of Aberrant Glycosylation and Its Mechanistic Causes in Colorectal Cancer Cells." *Journal of Proteome Research* 8 (6): 2990–3005. https://doi.org/10.1021/pr900092r.

Moore, Helen M., Andrea Kelly, Lisa M. McShane, and Jim Vaught. 2013. "Biospecimen Reporting for Improved Study Quality (BRISQ)." *Transfusion* 53 (7). https://doi.org/10.1111/trf.12281.

Mortazavi, Hamed, Maryam Baharvand, and Masoumeh Mehdipour. 2014. "Oral Potentially Malignant Disorders: An Overview of More than 20 Entities." *Journal of Dental Research, Dental Clinics, Dental Prospects* 8 (1): 6–14. https://doi.org/10.5681/joddd.2014.002.

Müller-Tidow, Carsten, Hans Ulrich Klein, Antje Hascher, Fabienne Isken, Lara Tickenbrock, Nils Thoennissen, Shuchi Agrawal-Singh, et al. 2010. "Profiling of Histone H3 Lysine 9 Trimethylation Levels Predicts Transcription Factor Activity and Survival in Acute Myeloid Leukemia." *Blood* 116 (18): 3564–71. https://doi.org/10.1182/blood-2009-09-240978.

Murali, Abitha, K. R. Nalinakumari, Shaji Thomas, and S. Kannan. 2014. "Association of Single Nucleotide Polymorphisms in Cell Cycle Regulatory Genes with Oral Cancer Susceptibility." *British Journal of Oral and Maxillofacial Surgery* 52 (7): 652–58. https://doi.org/10.1016/j.bjoms.2014.05.010.

Nakamura, Jun, Tomokazu Tanaka, Yoshihiko Kitajima, Hirokazu Noshiro, and Kohji Miyazaki. 2014. "Methylation-Mediated Gene Silencing as Biomarkers of Gastric Cancer: A Review." *World Journal of Gastroenterology*. WJG Press. https://doi.org/10.3748/wjg.v20.i34.11991.

Nakamura, Kodai, Naomi Hiyake, Tomofumi Hamada, Seiya Yokoyama, Kazuki Mori, Kouta Yamashiro, Mahiro Beppu, Yasuaki Sagara, Yoshiaki Sagara, and Tsuyoshi Sugiura. 2021. "Circulating MicroRNA Panel as a Potential Novel Biomarker for Oral Squamous Cell Carcinoma Diagnosis." *Cancers* 13 (3): 1–14. https://doi.org/10.3390/cancers13030449.

Narod, S. A., A. Seth, and R. Nam. 2008. "Fusion in the ETS Gene Family and Prostate Cancer." *British Journal of Cancer*. Nature Publishing Group. https://doi.org/10.1038/sj.bjc.6604558.

Németh, Christopher G., Christoph Röcken, Reiner Siebert, Jörg Wiltfang, Ole Ammerpohl, and Volker Gassling. 2019. "Recurrent Chromosomal and Epigenetic Alterations in Oral Squamous Cell Carcinoma and Its Putative Premalignant Condition Oral Lichen Planus." *PLoS ONE* 14 (4). https://doi.org/10.1371/journal.pone.0215055.

Neves Drummond, Sérgio, Ricardo Santiago Gomez, Júlio Carlos Motta Noronha, Isabela Almeida Pordeus, Alvimar Afonso Barbosa, and Luiz De Marco. 2005. "Association between GSTT-1 Gene Deletion and the Susceptibility to Oral Squamous Cell Carcinoma in Cigarette-Smoking Subjects." *Oral Oncology* 41 (5): 515–19. https://doi.org/10.1016/j.oraloncology.2004.12.014.

Niu, Yu Ming, Xin Ya Du, Heng Xing Cai, Chao Zhang, Rui Xia Yuan, Xian Tao Zeng, and Jie Luo. 2015. "Increased Risks between Interleukin-10 Gene Polymorphisms and Haplotype and Head and Neck Cancer: A Meta-Analysis." *Scientific Reports* 5. https://doi.org/10.1038/srep17149.

"No Title." n.d. https://next.cancer.gov/developmentresources/pd_biomarker.

Numasawa, Hideyuki, Nobuharu Yamamoto, Akira Katakura, and Takahiko Shibahara. 2005. "Loss of Heterozygosity and Microsatellite Instability on Chromosome 2q in Human Oral Squamous Cell Carcinoma." *The Bulletin of Tokyo Dental College* 46 (1–2): 17–25. https://doi.org/10.2209/tdcpublication.46.17.

Núñez, Cristina. 2019. "Blood-Based Protein Biomarkers in Breast Cancer." *Clinica Chimica Acta*. Elsevier B.V. https://doi.org/10.1016/j.cca.2018.12.028.

Obaidul, Mohammad, Hoque Johns, Hopkins Medicine, Qinghua Feng, Stephen E Hawes, Mohammad O Hoque, Papa Toure, et al. 2006. "Detection of Aberrant Methylation of Four Genes in Plasma DNA for the Detection of Breast Cancer." *Article in Journal of Clinical Oncology* 24: 4262–69. https://doi.org/10.1200/JCO.2005.01.3516.

Oh, Su Young, Sung-Min Kang, Soo Hyun Kang, Heon-Jin Lee, Tae-Geon Kwon, Jin-Wook Kim, Sung-Tak Lee, So-Young Choi, and Su-Hyung Hong. 2020. "Potential Salivary MRNA Biomarkers for Early Detection of Oral Cancer." *Journal of Clinical Medicine* 9 (1): 243. https://doi.org/10.3390/jcm9010243.

Oliveira-Costa, Joao Paulo, Alex Fiorini de Carvalho, Giorgia Gobbi da Silveira, Peter Amaya, Yongqi Wu, Kyoung Joo Jenny Park, Mabel Pinilla Gigliola, et al. 2015. "Gene Expression Patterns through Oral Squamous Cell Carcinoma Development: PD-L1 Expression in Primary Tumor and Circulating Tumor Cells." *Oncotarget* 6 (25): 20902–20. https://doi.org/10.18632/oncotarget.3939.

Oliveira Ribeiro, Artur de, Luiz Carlos Ferreira da Silva, and Paulo Ricardo Saquete Martins-Filho. 2014. "Prevalence of and Risk Factors for Actinic Cheilitis in Brazilian Fishermen and Women." *International Journal of Dermatology* 53 (11): 1370–76. https://doi.org/10.1111/ijd.12526.

Osada, Hirotaka, Yoshio Tatematsu, Hiroko Saito, Yasushi Yatabe, Tetsuya Mitsudomi, and Takashi Takahashi. 2004. "Reduced Expression of Class II Histone Deacetylase Genes Is Associated with Poor Prognosis in Lung Cancer Patients." *International Journal of Cancer* 112 (1): 26–32. https://doi.org/10.1002/ijc.20395.

Pan, Tao, Yong guo Li, Ke yi Li, Cheng Chen, Kai Xu, Dao ying Yuan, Bo Zou, and Zhen Meng. 2020. "Identification of a Novel Fusion Gene, TRIM52-RACK1, in Oral Squamous Cell Carcinoma." *Molecular and Cellular Probes* 52. https://doi.org/10.1016/j.mcp.2020.101568.

Panda, Swagatika, VT Beena, Kanaram Choudhary, KR Nalinakumari, Moinak Banerjee, R Sivakumar, and Sanish Sathyan. 2015. "Microsatellite Instability in D2S123 Flanking the HMSH2 Gene in Oral Squamous Cell Carcinoma in South India." *Clinical Cancer Investigation Journal* 4 (1): 22. https://doi.org/10.4103/2278-0513.149031.

Pang, Qianqian, Jiaxin Ge, Yongfu Shao, Weiliang Sun, Haojun Song, Tian Xia, Bingxiu Xiao, and Junming Guo. 2014. "Increased Expression of Long Intergenic Non-Coding RNA LINC00152 in Gastric Cancer and Its Clinical Significance." *Tumor Biology* 35 (6): 5441–47. https://doi.org/10.1007/s13277-014-1709-3.

Papanikolaou, Vasileios S., Efthymios Kyrodimos, Evangelos Tsiambas, Evangelos Giotakis, Amanta Psyrri, Vasileios Ragos, and Aristeidis

Chrysovergis. 2018. "Chromosomal Instability in Oral Squamous Cell Carcinoma." *Journal of B.U.ON.* 23 (6): 1580–82.

Payne, Shannon R., Jurgen Serth, Martin Schostak, Jorn Kamradt, Arne Strauss, Paul Thelen, Fabian Model, et al. 2009. "DNA Methylation Biomarkers of Prostate Cancer: Confirmation of Candidates and Evidence Urine Is the Most Sensitive Body Fluid for Non-Invasive Detection." *Prostate* 69 (12): 1257–69. https://doi.org/10.1002/pros.20967.

Peng, Cheng, Yanshuo Ye, Zhanpeng Wang, Lianyue Guan, Suriguga Bao, Bo Li, and Wei Li. 2019. "Circulating MicroRNAs for the Diagnosis of Hepatocellular Carcinoma." *Digestive and Liver Disease*. Elsevier B.V. https://doi.org/10.1016/j.dld.2018.12.011.

Peng, Guiyong, Qinglin Long, Yuwei Wu, Jingjing Zhao, Lei Chen, and Xianghong Li. 2011. "Evaluation of Double Vital Staining with Lugol's Iodine and Methylene Blue in Diagnosing Superficial Esophageal Lesions." *Scandinavian Journal of Gastroenterology* 46 (4): 406–13. https://doi.org/10.3109/00365521.2010.545829.

Petersen, Poul Erik. 2009. "Oral Cancer Prevention and Control - The Approach of the World Health Organization." *Oral Oncology*. https://doi.org/10.1016/j.oraloncology.2008.05.023.

Powlesland, Alex S., Paul G. Hitchen, Simon Parry, Sarah A. Graham, Maria Marcela Barrio, Maria Teresa Elola, José Mordoh, Anne Dell, Kurt Drickamer, and Maureen E. Taylor. 2009. "Targeted Glycoproteomic Identification of Cancer Cell Glycosylation." *Glycobiology* 19 (8): 899–909. https://doi.org/10.1093/glycob/cwp065.

Powrózek, T., P. Krawczyk, M. Nicoś, B. Kuźnar-Kamińska, H. Batura-Gabryel, and J. Milanowski. 2016. "Methylation of the DCLK1 Promoter Region in Circulating Free DNA and Its Prognostic Value in Lung Cancer Patients." *Clinical and Translational Oncology* 18 (4): 398–404. https://doi.org/10.1007/s12094-015-1382-z.

Preston, R Julian. 2006. "The Use of Biomarkers in Cancer Risk Assessment." *Epidemiology* 17 (Suppl): S25–26. https://doi.org/10.1097/00001648-200611001-00021.

Principe, Simona, Angela Bik Yu Hui, Jeff Bruce, Ankit Sinha, Fei Fei Liu, and Thomas Kislinger. 2013. "Tumor-Derived Exosomes and Microvesicles in Head and Neck Cancer: Implications for Tumor Biology and Biomarker Discovery." *Proteomics* 13 (10–11): 1608–23. https://doi.org/10.1002/pmic.201200533.

Qian, Ke, Gao Liu, Zhonghua Tang, Yibo Hu, Yu Fang, Zonglin Chen, and Xundi Xu. 2017. "The Long Non-Coding RNA NEAT1 Interacted with MiR-101 Modulates Breast Cancer Growth by Targeting EZH2." *Archives of Biochemistry and Biophysics* 615 (February): 1–9. https://doi.org/10.1016/j.abb.2016.12.011.

Ramalho-Carvalho, João, Rui Henrique, and Carmen Jerónimo. 2018. "Methylation-Specific PCR." In *Methods in Molecular Biology*, 1708:447–72. Humana Press Inc. https://doi.org/10.1007/978-1-4939-7481-8_23.

Rana, Majeed, Antonia Zapf, Marco Kuehle, Nils Claudius Gellrich, and André M. Eckardt. 2012. "Clinical Evaluation of an Autofluorescence Diagnostic Device for Oral Cancer Detection: A Prospective Randomized Diagnostic Study." *European Journal of Cancer Prevention* 21 (5): 460–66. https://doi.org/10.1097/CEJ.0b013e32834fdb6d.

Ransohoff, David F., and Margaret L. Gourlay. 2010. "Sources of Bias in Specimens for Research about Molecular Markers for Cancer." *Journal of Clinical Oncology* 28 (4): 698–704. https://doi.org/10.1200/JCO.2009.25.6065.

Rao, Umadevi Krishna Mohan, Rooban Thavarajah, Elizabeth Joshua, and Kannan Ranganathan. 2018. "Loss of Heterozygosity as a Marker to Predict Progression of Oral Epithelial Dysplasia to Oral Squamous Cell Carcinoma." *Journal of Oral and Maxillofacial Pathology* 22 (2): 155–60. https://doi.org/10.4103/jomfp.JOMFP_151_18.

Ren, Wenhao, Cui Qiang, Ling Gao, Shao Ming Li, Lin Mei Zhang, Xiao Long Wang, Jian Wei Dong, Cheng Chen, Chang Yang Liu, and Ke Qian Zhi. 2014. "Circulating MicroRNA-21 (MIR-21) and Phosphatase and Tensin Homolog (PTEN) Are Promising Novel Biomarkers for

Detection of Oral Squamous Cell Carcinoma." *Biomarkers* 19 (7): 590–96. https://doi.org/10.3109/1354750X.2014.955059.

Rethman, Michael P., William Carpenter, Ezra E.W. Cohen, Joel Epstein, Caswell A. Evans, Catherine M. Flalfz, Frank J. Graham, et al. 2010. "Evidence-Based Clinical Recommendations Regarding Screening for Oral Squamous Cell Carcinomas." *Journal of the American Dental Association* 141 (5): 509–20. https://doi.org/10.14219/jada.archive.2010.0223.

Rettori, Marianna Marconato, Ana Carolina De carvalho, Ana Luiza Bomfim longo, Cleyton Zanardo De oliveira, Luiz Paulo Kowalski, Andre Lopes Carvalho, and Andre Luiz Vettore. 2013. "Prognostic Significance of TIMP3 Hypermethylation in Post-Treatment Salivary Rinse from Head and Neck Squamous Cell Carcinoma Patients." *Carcinogenesis* 34 (1): 20–27. https://doi.org/10.1093/carcin/bgs311.

Rivera, César, Ana Karina Oliveira, Rute Alves Pereira Costa, Tatiane De Rossi, and Adriana Franco Paes Leme. 2017. "Prognostic Biomarkers in Oral Squamous Cell Carcinoma: A Systematic Review." *Oral Oncology* 72: 38–47. https://doi.org/10.1016/j.oraloncology.2017.07.003.

Romani, Chiara, Elisa Salviato, Alberto Paderno, Laura Zanotti, Antonella Ravaggi, Alberto Deganello, Giulia Berretti, et al. 2021. "Genome-Wide Study of Salivary MiRNAs Identifies MiR-423-5p as Promising Diagnostic and Prognostic Biomarker in Oral Squamous Cell Carcinoma." *Theranostics* 11 (6): 2987–99. https://doi.org/10.7150/THNO.45157.

Rosenberg, Dara, and Shan Cretin. 1989. "Use of Meta-Analysis to Evaluate Tolonium Chloride in Oral Cancer Screening." *Oral Surgery, Oral Medicine, Oral Pathology* 67 (5): 621–27. https://doi.org/10.1016/0030-4220(89)90286-7.

Rosenfeld, Nitzan, Ranit Aharonov, Eti Meiri, Shai Rosenwald, Yael Spector, Merav Zepeniuk, Hila Benjamin, et al. 2008. "MicroRNAs Accurately Identify Cancer Tissue Origin." *Nature Biotechnology* 26 (4): 462–69. https://doi.org/10.1038/nbt1392.

Rossi, Marianna Nicoletta, and Fabrizio Antonangeli. 2014. "LncRNAs: New Players in Apoptosis Control." *International Journal of Cell Biology*. https://doi.org/10.1155/2014/473857.

Ruberg, Stephen J., and Lei Shen. 2015. "Personalized Medicine: Four Perspectives of Tailored Medicine." *Statistics in Biopharmaceutical Research* 7 (3): 214–29. https://doi.org/10.1080/19466315.2015.1059354.

Sakuma, Takumi, Katsuhiro Uzawa, Takeshi Onda, Masashi Shiiba, Hidetaka Yokoe, Takahiko Shibahara, and Hideki Tanzawa. 2006. "Aberrant Expression of Histone Deacetylase 6 in Oral Squamous Cell Carcinoma." *International Journal of Oncology* 29 (1): 117–24. https://doi.org/10.3892/ijo.29.1.117.

Saldova, Radka, Mark R. Wormald, Raymond A. Dwek, and Pauline M. Rudd. 2008. "Glycosylation Changes on Serum Glycoproteins in Ovarian Cancer May Contribute to Disease Pathogenesis." *Disease Markers* 25 (4–5): 219–32. https://doi.org/10.1155/2008/601583.

Sankaranarayanan, Rengaswamy, Ramani Wesley, Somanathan Thara, Namrata Dhakad, Bharathykutty Chandralekha, Paul Sebastian, K. Chithrathara, Donald Maxwell Parkin, and Madhavan Krishnan Nair. 2003. "Test Characteristics of Visual Inspection with 4% Acetic Acid (VIA) and Lugol's Iodine (VILI) in Cervical Cancer Screening in Kerala, India." *International Journal of Cancer* 106 (3): 404–8. https://doi.org/10.1002/ijc.11245.

Sarker, Debashis, and Paul Workman. 2006. "Pharmacodynamic Biomarkers for Molecular Cancer Therapeutics." *Advances in Cancer Research* 96: 213–68. https://doi.org/10.1016/S0065-230X(06)96008-4.

Sasaki, Hidefumi, Satoru Moriyama, Yoshiaki Nakashima, Yoshihiro Kobayashi, Masanobu Kiriyama, Ichiro Fukai, Yosuke Yamakawa, and Yoshitaka Fujii. 2004. "Histone Deacetylase 1 MRNA Expression in Lung Cancer." *Lung Cancer* 46 (2): 171–78. https://doi.org/10.1016/j.lungcan.2004.03.021.

Scheifele, Christian, Andrea Maria Schmidt-Westhausen, Thomas Dietrich, and Peter A. Reichart. 2004. "The Sensitivity and Specificity of the

OralCDx Technique: Evaluation of 103 Cases." *Oral Oncology* 40 (8): 824–28. https://doi.org/10.1016/j.oraloncology.2004.02.004.

Schubert, Mark M., and Maria Elvira Pizzigatti Correa. 2008. "Oral Graft-Versus-Host Disease." *Dental Clinics of North America* 52 (1): 79–109. https://doi.org/10.1016/j.cden.2007.10.004.

Schwarzenbach, Heidi, Naohiro Nishida, George A. Calin, and Klaus Pantel. 2014. "Clinical Relevance of Circulating Cell-Free MicroRNAs in Cancer." *Nature Reviews Clinical Oncology 2014 11:3* 11 (3): 145–56. https://doi.org/10.1038/nrclinonc.2014.5.

Sciubba, James J. 1999. "Improving Detection of Precancerous and Cancerous Oral Lesions: Computer-Assisted Analysis of the Oral Brush Biopsy." *Journal of the American Dental Association* 130 (10): 1445–57. https://doi.org/10.14219/jada.archive.1999.0055.

Sechidis, Konstantinos, Konstantinos Papangelou, Paul D. Metcalfe, David Svensson, James Weatherall, and Gavin Brown. 2018. "Distinguishing Prognostic and Predictive Biomarkers: An Information Theoretic Approach." *Bioinformatics* 34 (19): 3365–76. https://doi.org/10.1093/bioinformatics/bty357.

Seki, Sachiko, Mutsunori Fujiwara, Masaaki Matsuura, Shuichi Fujita, Hisazumi Ikeda, Izumi Asahina, and Tohru Ikeda. 2011. "Prediction of Outcome of Patients with Oral Squamous Cell Carcinoma Using Vascular Invasion and the Strongly Positive Expression of Vascular Endothelial Growth Factors." *Oral Oncology* 47 (7): 588–93. https://doi.org/10.1016/j.oraloncology.2011.04.013.

Shah, Neha, Jay Gopal Ray, Sanchita Kundu, and Divesh Sardana. 2017. "Surgical Management of Chronic Hyperplastic Candidiasis Refractory to Systemic Antifungal Treatment." *Journal of Laboratory Physicians* 9 (02): 136–39. https://doi.org/10.4103/0974-2727.199622.

Shao, Yongfu, Jinyun Li, Rongdan Lu, Tianwen Li, Yunben Yang, Bingxiu Xiao, and Junming Guo. 2017. "Global Circular RNA Expression Profile of Human Gastric Cancer and Its Clinical Significance." *Cancer Medicine* 6 (6): 1173–80. https://doi.org/10.1002/cam4.1055.

Shao, Yongfu, Meng Ye, Xiaoming Jiang, Weiliang Sun, Xiaoyun Ding, Zhong Liu, Guoliang Ye, Xinjun Zhang, Bingxiu Xiao, and Junming

Guo. 2014. "Gastric Juice Long Noncoding RNA Used as a Tumor Marker for Screening Gastric Cancer." *Cancer* 120 (21): 3320–28. https://doi.org/10.1002/cncr.28882.

Singh, Neetu, Dinesh Kumar Sahu, Ratnesh Kumar Tripathi, Archana Mishra, Hari Shyam, Pratap Shankar, Mayank Jain, et al. 2020. "Differentially Expressed Full-Length, Fusion and Novel Isoforms Transcripts-Based Signature of Well-Differentiated Keratinized Oral Squamous Cell Carcinoma." *Oncotarget* 11 (34): 3227–43. https://doi.org/10.18632/oncotarget.27693.

Singh, Pooja, Anand Narain Srivastava, Rolee Sharma, Saboor Mateen, Bharat Shukla, Alok Singh, and Siddhartha Chandel. 2018. "Circulating MicroRNA-21 Expression as a Novel Serum Biomarker for Oral Sub-Mucous Fibrosis and Oral Squamous Cell Carcinoma." *Asian Pacific Journal of Cancer Prevention* 19 (4): 1053–58. https://doi.org/10.22034/APJCP.2018.19.4.1053.

Siow, M. Y., L. P. Karen Ng, V. K. Vincent Chong, M. Jamaludin, M. T. Abraham, Z. A. Abdul Rahman, T. G. Kallarakkal, Y. H. Yang, S. C. Cheong, and R. B. Zain. 2014. "Dysregulation of MiR-31 and MiR-375 Expression Is Associated with Clinical Outcomes in Oral Carcinoma." *Oral Diseases* 20 (4): 345–51. https://doi.org/10.1111/odi.12118.

Smadbeck, James, Jess F. Peterson, Kathryn E. Pearce, Beth A. Pitel, Andrea Lebron Figueroa, Michael Timm, A. Dragan Jevremovic, et al. 2019. "Mate Pair Sequencing Outperforms Fluorescence in Situ Hybridization in the Genomic Characterization of Multiple Myeloma." *Blood Cancer Journal* 9 (12): 103. https://doi.org/10.1038/s41408-019-0255-z.

Song, Chun Jiao, Huan Chen, Li Zhong Chen, Guo Mei Ru, Jian Jun Guo, and Qian Nan Ding. 2018. "The Potential of MicroRNAs as Human Prostate Cancer Biomarkers: A Meta-Analysis of Related Studies." *Journal of Cellular Biochemistry* 119 (3): 2763–86. https://doi.org/10.1002/jcb.26445.

Song, Joon Seon, Yong Seok Kim, Dong Kwan Kim, Sung il Park, and Se Jin Jang. 2012. "Global Histone Modification Pattern Associated with Recurrence and Disease-Free Survival in Non-Small Cell Lung Cancer

Patients." *Pathology International* 62 (3): 182–90. https://doi.org/10.1111/j.1440-1827.2011.02776.x.

Sowmya, SV, RoopaS Rao, and Kavitha Prasad. 2020. "Prediction of Metastasis in Oral Squamous Cell Carcinoma through Phenotypic Evaluation and Gene Expression of E-Cadherin, β-Catenin, Matrix Metalloproteinase-2, and Matrix Metalloproteinase-9 Biomarkers with Clinical Correlation." *Journal of Carcinogenesis* 19 (1): 8. https://doi.org/10.4103/jcar.jcar_8_20.

Stojanovic, Jovana, Alessia Tognetto, Danilo Francesco Tiziano, Emanuele Leoncini, Brunella Posteraro, Roberta Pastorino, and Stefania Boccia. 2019. "MicroRNAs Expression Profiles as Diagnostic Biomarkers of Gastric Cancer: A Systematic Literature Review." *Biomarkers*. Taylor and Francis Ltd. https://doi.org/10.1080/1354750X.2018.1539765.

Strzelczyk, Joanna Katarzyna, Lukasz Krakowczyk, and Aleksander Jerzy Owczarek. 2018. "Aberrant DNA Methylation of the P16, APC, MGMT, TIMP3 and CDH1 Gene Promoters in Tumours and the Surgical Margins of Patients with Oral Cavity Cancer." *Journal of Cancer* 9 (11): 1896–1904. https://doi.org/10.7150/jca.24477.

Su, Chen, Hanwei Li, Zheng Peng, Dong Ke, Hanjiang Fu, and Xiaofei Zheng. 2019. "Identification of Plasma RGS18 and PPBP MRNAs as Potential Biomarkers for Gastric Cancer Using Transcriptome Arrays." *Oncology Letters* 17 (1): 247–55. https://doi.org/10.3892/ol.2018.9608.

Su, Xiaogang, Tianni Zhou, Xin Yan, Juanjuan Fan, and Song Yang. 2008. "Interaction Trees with Censored Survival Data." *International Journal of Biostatistics* 4 (1). https://doi.org/10.2202/1557-4679.1071.

Sukhija, Hemani, Rajkumar Krishnan, N. Balachander, Karthik Raghavendhar, Ramya Ramadoss, and Sukanta Sen. 2015. "C-Deletion in Exon 4 Codon 63 of P53 Gene as a Molecular Marker for Oral Squamous Cell Carcinoma: A Preliminary Study." *Contemporary Clinical Dentistry* 6: S227–34. https://doi.org/10.4103/0976-237X.166840.

Sun, Guan, Ying Cao, Peibei Wang, Hongmao Song, Tongwu Bie, Min Li, and De Huai. 2018. "MiR-200b-3p in Plasma Is a Potential Diagnostic

Biomarker in Oral Squamous Cell Carcinoma." *Biomarkers* 23 (2): 137–41. https://doi.org/10.1080/1354750X.2017.1289241.

Sun, Shuai, Bowen Li, Yufan Wang, Xiang Li, Panpan Wang, Feng Wang, Wei Zhang, and Hongyu Yang. 2018. "Clinical Significance of the Decreased Expression of Hsa_circ_001242 in Oral Squamous Cell Carcinoma." *Disease Markers* 2018. https://doi.org/10.1155/2018/6514795.

Svoboda, M., J. Slyskova, M. Schneiderova, P. Makovicky, L. Bielik, M. Levy, L. Lipska, et al. 2014. "HOTAIR Long Non-Coding RNA Is a Negative Prognostic Factor Not Only in Primary Tumors, but Also in the Blood of Colorectal Cancer Patients." *Carcinogenesis* 35 (7): 1510–15. https://doi.org/10.1093/carcin/bgu055.

Taioli, Emanuela, Camille Ragin, Xiao hong Wang, Jiangying Chen, Scott M. Langevin, Ashley R. Brown, Susanne M. Gollin, Seymour Garte, and Robert W. Sobol. 2009. "Recurrence in Oral and Pharyngeal Cancer Is Associated with Quantitative MGMT Promoter Methylation." *BMC Cancer* 9 (1): 354. https://doi.org/10.1186/1471-2407-9-354.

Tan, Shuangyan, Qiheng Gou, Wenchen Pu, Chenglin Guo, Yun Yang, Ke Wu, Yaxin Liu, Lunxu Liu, Yu Quan Wei, and Yong Peng. 2018. "Circular RNA F-CircEA Produced from EML4-ALK Fusion Gene as a Novel Liquid Biopsy Biomarker for Non-Small Cell Lung Cancer." *Cell Research*. Nature Publishing Group. https://doi.org/10.1038/s41422-018-0033-7.

Tang, Haikuo, Zhiyuan Wu, Jianping Zhang, and Bing Su. 2013. "Salivary LncRNA as a Potential Marker for Oral Squamous Cell Carcinoma Diagnosis." *Molecular Medicine Reports* 7 (3): 761–66. https://doi.org/10.3892/mmr.2012.1254.

Tang, Junwei, Runqiu Jiang, Lei Deng, Xudong Zhang, Ke Wang, and Beicheng Sun. 2015. "Circulation Long Non-Coding RNAs Act as Biomarkers for Predicting Tumorigenesis and Metastasis in Hepatocellular Carcinoma." *Oncotarget* 6 (6): 4505–15. https://doi.org/10.18632/oncotarget.2934.

Tani, Nobuyuki, Daisuke Ichikawa, Daito Ikoma, Haruhisa Tomita, Soujin Sai, Hisashi Ikoma, Kazuma Okamoto, et al. 2007. "Circulating Cell-

Free MRNA in Plasma as a Tumor Marker for Patients with Primary and Recurrent Gastric Cancer." *Anticancer Research* 27 (2).

Teutsch, Steven M., Linda A. Bradley, Glenn E. Palomaki, James E. Haddow, Margaret Piper, Ned Calonge, W. David Dotson, Michael P. Douglas, and Alfred O. Berg. 2010. "The Evaluation of Genomic Applications in Practice and Prevention (EGAPP) Initiative: Methods of the EGAPP Working Group." *Human Genome Epidemiology: Building the Evidence for Using Genetic Information to Improve Health and Prevent Disease: Second Edition.* https://doi.org/10.1093/acprof:oso/9780195398441.003.0023.

Thompson, Lester D.R. 2006. "World Health Organization Classification of Tumours: Pathology and Genetics of Head and Neck Tumours." *Ear, Nose and Throat Journal* 85 (2): 74. https://doi.org/10.1177/014556130608500201.

Tomlins, Scott A., Daniel R. Rhodes, Sven Perner, Saravana M. Dhanasekaran, Rohit Mehra, Xiao Wei Sun, Sooryanarayana Varambally, et al. 2005. "Recurrent Fusion of TMPRSS2 and ETS Transcription Factor Genes in Prostate Cancer." *Science* 310 (5748): 644–48. https://doi.org/10.1126/science.1117679.

Tong, Yu-Suo, Xiao-Wei Wang, Xi-Lei Zhou, Zi-Hao Liu, Tong-Xin Yang, Wei-Hong Shi, Hai-Wei Xie, Jin Lv, Qing-Quan Wu, and Xiu-Feng Cao. 2015. "Identification of the Long Non-Coding RNA POU3F3 in Plasma as a Novel Biomarker for Diagnosis of Esophageal Squamous Cell Carcinoma." *Molecular Cancer* 14 (1): 3. https://doi.org/10.1186/1476-4598-14-3.

Tost, Jörg, ed. 2018. *DNA Methylation Protocols*. Vol. 1708. Methods in Molecular Biology. New York, NY: Springer New York. https://doi.org/10.1007/978-1-4939-7481-8.

Tran, Anh Nhi, Fulya Taylan, Vasilios Zachariadis, Ingegerd Ivanov Öfverholm, Anna Lindstrand, Francesco Vezzi, Britta Lötstedt, et al. 2018. "High-Resolution Detection of Chromosomal Rearrangements in Leukemias through Mate Pair Whole Genome Sequencing." Edited by Obul Reddy Bandapalli. *PLoS ONE* 13 (3): e0193928. https://doi.org/10.1371/journal.pone.0193928.

Trivedi, T. I., R. A. Tankshali, J. V. Goswami, S. N. Shukla, P. M. Shah, and N. G. Shah. 2011. "Identification of Site-Specific Prognostic Biomarkers in Patients with Oral Squamous Cell Carcinoma." *Neoplasma* 58 (3): 217–26. https://doi.org/10.4149/neo_2011_03_217.

Tung, Chun Liang, Szu Ting Lin, Hsiu Chuan Chou, Yi Wen Chen, Hwan Chung Lin, Chung Liang Tung, Kao Jean Huang, Yi Ju Chen, Ying Ray Lee, and Hong Lin Chan. 2013. "Proteomics-Based Identification of Plasma Biomarkers in Oral Squamous Cell Carcinoma." *Journal of Pharmaceutical and Biomedical Analysis* 75: 7–17. https://doi.org/10.1016/j.jpba.2012.11.017.

Tzao, Ching, Ho Jui Tung, Jong Shiaw Jin, Guang Huan Sun, Han Shui Hsu, Ban Hen Chen, Cheng Ping Yu, and Shih Chun Lee. 2009. "Prognostic Significance of Global Histone Modifications in Resected Squamous Cell Carcinoma of the Esophagus." *Modern Pathology* 22 (2): 252–60. https://doi.org/10.1038/modpathol.2008.172.

Umare, Vinod, Vandana Pradhan, Sneha Dadheech, Anjali Rajadhyaksha, Kanjaksha Ghosh, and Anita Nadkarni. 2020. "Clinical Implications of IL-10 Promoter Polymorphisms on Disease Susceptibility in Indian SLE Patients." *Lupus* 29 (6): 587–98. https://doi.org/10.1177/0961203320913619.

Vadas, Mathew, Pu Xia, Geoff McCaughan, and Jennifer Gamble. 2008. "The Role of Sphingosine Kinase 1 in Cancer: Oncogene or Non-Oncogene Addiction?" *Biochimica et Biophysica Acta - Molecular and Cell Biology of Lipids* 1781 (9): 442–47. https://doi.org/10.1016/j.bbalip.2008.06.007.

Valadi, Hadi, Karin Ekström, Apostolos Bossios, Margareta Sjöstrand, James J. Lee, and Jan O. Lötvall. 2007. "Exosome-Mediated Transfer of MRNAs and MicroRNAs Is a Novel Mechanism of Genetic Exchange between Cells." *Nature Cell Biology* 9 (6): 654–59. https://doi.org/10.1038/ncb1596.

Varshitha, A. 2015. "Prevalence of Oral Cancer in India." *Journal of Pharmaceutical Sciences and Research.*

Vinayanuwattikun, Chanida, Virote Sriuranpong, Suebpong Tanasanvimon, Poonchavist Chantranuwat, and Apiwat Mutirangura. 2011. "Epithelial-

Specific Methylation Marker: A Potential Plasma Biomarker in Advanced Non-Small Cell Lung Cancer." *Journal of Thoracic Oncology* 6 (11): 1818–25. https://doi.org/10.1097/JTO.0b013e318226b46f.

Vincent-Chong, Vui King, Iman Salahshourifar, Kar Mun Woo, Arif Anwar, Rozaimi Razali, Ranganath Gudimella, Zainal Ariff Abdul Rahman, et al. 2017. "Genome Wide Profiling in Oral Squamous Cell Carcinoma Identifies a Four Genetic Marker Signature of Prognostic Significance." Edited by Xuefeng Liu. *PLoS ONE* 12 (4): e0174865. https://doi.org/10.1371/journal.pone.0174865.

Viswanathan, Muthusamy, Nobuo Tsuchida, and Govindaswamy Shanmugam. 2003. "Promoter Hypermethylation Profile of Tumor-Associated Genes P16, P15, HMLH1, MGMT and E-Cadherin in Oral Squamous Cell Carcinoma." *International Journal of Cancer* 105 (1): 41–46. https://doi.org/10.1002/ijc.11028.

Waidely, Eric, Abdul Rahman Obaid Al-Yuobi, A. S. Bashammakh, Mohammad S. El-Shahawi, and Roger M. Leblanc. 2016. "Serum Protein Biomarkers Relevant to Hepatocellular Carcinoma and Their Detection." *Analyst.* Royal Society of Chemistry. https://doi.org/10.1039/c5an01884f.

Waldron, Charles A., and William G. Shafer. 1975. "Leukoplakia Revisited. A Clinicopathologic Study 3256 Oral Leukoplakias." *Cancer* 36 (4): 1386–92. https://doi.org/10.1002/1097-0142(197510)36:4<1386::AID-CNCR2820360430>3.0.CO;2-7.

Wang, Bo, Shu Zhang, Kai Yue, and Xu Dong Wang. 2013. "The Recurrence and Survival of Oral Squamous Cell Carcinoma: A Report of 275 Cases." *Chinese Journal of Cancer* 32 (11): 614–18. https://doi.org/10.5732/cjc.012.10219.

Wang, Ruinan, Yao Yuan, Yuqiao Zhou, Dunfang Zhang, Lewei Zhang, Xin Zeng, Ning Ji, et al. 2018. "Screening Diagnostic Biomarkers of OSCC via an LCM-Based Proteomic Approach." *Oncology Reports* 40 (4): 2088–96. https://doi.org/10.3892/or.2018.6610.

Wang, Wenjian, Xiaotian He, Zehua Zheng, Xiaofan Ma, Xueting Hu, Duoguang Wu, and Minghui Wang. 2017. "Serum HOTAIR as a Novel

Diagnostic Biomarker for Esophageal Squamous Cell Carcinoma." *Molecular Cancer* 16 (1). https://doi.org/10.1186/s12943-017-0643-6.

Wang, Yun, Lin Lin, Hao Xu, Taiwen Li, Yu Zhou, Hongxia Dan, Lu Jiang, et al. 2015. "Genetic Variants in AKT1 Gene Were Associated with Risk and Survival of OSCC in Chinese Han Population." *Journal of Oral Pathology and Medicine* 44 (1): 45–50. https://doi.org/10.1111/jop.12211.

Wang, Yun, Chongkui Sun, Taiwen Li, Hao Xu, Yu Zhou, Hongxia Dan, Lu Jiang, et al. 2014. "Integrative Approach Detected Association between Genetic Variants of MicroRNA Binding Sites of TLRs Pathway Genes and OSCC Susceptibility in Chinese Han Population." Edited by Sevtap Savas. *PLoS ONE* 9 (7): e101695. https://doi.org/10.1371/journal.pone.0101695.

Wang, Yuxuan, Simeon Springer, Carolyn L. Mulvey, Natalie Silliman, Joy Schaefer, Mark Sausen, Nathan James, et al. 2015. "Detection of Somatic Mutations and HPV in the Saliva and Plasma of Patients with Head and Neck Squamous Cell Carcinomas." *Science Translational Medicine* 7 (293). https://doi.org/10.1126/scitranslmed.aaa8507.

Wang, Zihong, Jing Tang, Yufan Wang, Shuai Sun, Yuling Chen, Yuehong Shen, and Hong Yu Yang. 2019. "Circular RNA Hsa_circ_009755 Downregulation Correlates with Clinicopathology in Oral Squamous Cell Carcinoma." *OncoTargets and Therapy* 12 (May): 4025–31. https://doi.org/10.2147/OTT.S196618.

Warnakulasuriya, S. 1987. "Semi-Quantitative Clinical Description of Oral Submucous Fibrosis." *Annals of Dentistry* 46 (2): 18–21.

Warnakulasuriya, Saman. 2018. "Clinical Features and Presentation of Oral Potentially Malignant Disorders." *Oral Surgery, Oral Medicine, Oral Pathology and Oral Radiology* 125 (6): 582–90. https://doi.org/10.1016/j.oooo.2018.03.011.

Wei, Hui, Kang Yu, Yongheng Liu, Lili Li, and Guowen Wang. 2020. "Tumor Expression of MiR-448 Is a Prognostic Marker in Oral Squamous Cell Carcinoma." *BMC Cancer* 20 (1). https://doi.org/10.1186/s12885-020-07243-z.

Weichert, Wilko, Annika Röske, Volker Gekeler, Thomas Beckers, Matthias PA Ebert, Matthias Pross, Manfred Dietel, Carsten Denkert, and Christoph Röcken. 2008. "Association of Patterns of Class I Histone Deacetylase Expression with Patient Prognosis in Gastric Cancer: A Retrospective Analysis." *The Lancet Oncology* 9 (2): 139–48. https://doi.org/10.1016/S1470-2045(08)70004-4.

Weichert, Wilko, Annika Röske, Silvia Niesporek, Aurelia Noske, Ann Christin Buckendahl, Manfred Dietel, Volker Gekeler, Markus Boehm, Thomas Beckers, and Carsten Denkert. 2008. "Class I Histone Deacetylase Expression Has Independent Prognostic Impact in Human Colorectal Cancer: Specific Role of Class I Histone Deacetylases in Vitro and in Vivo." *Clinical Cancer Research* 14 (6): 1669–77. https://doi.org/10.1158/1078-0432.CCR-07-0990.

Weng, C. J., Y. H. Hsieh, M. K. Chen, C. M. Tsai, C. W. Lin, and S. F. Yang. 2012. "Survivin SNP-Carcinogen Interactions in Oral Cancer." *Journal of Dental Research* 91 (4): 358–63. https://doi.org/10.1177/0022034512438402.

Weng, Wenhao, Qing Wei, Shusuke Toden, Kazuhiro Yoshida, Takeshi Nagasaka, Toshiyoshi Fujiwara, Sanjun Cai, Huanlong Qin, Yanlei Ma, and Ajay Goel. 2017. "Circular RNA CiRS-7 — A Promising Prognostic Biomarker and a Potential Therapeutic Target in Colorectal Cancer." *Clinical Cancer Research* 23 (14): 3918–28. https://doi.org/10.1158/1078-0432.CCR-16-2541.

Werbrouck, Joke, Kim De Ruyck, Fréderic Duprez, Marc Van Eijkeren, Ernst Rietzschel, Sofie Bekaert, Anne Vral, Wilfried De Neve, and Hubert Thierens. 2008. "Single-Nucleotide Polymorphisms in DNA Double-Strand Break Repair Genes: Association with Head and Neck Cancer and Interaction with Tobacco Use and Alcohol Consumption." *Mutation Research - Genetic Toxicology and Environmental Mutagenesis* 656 (1–2): 74–81. https://doi.org/10.1016/j.mrgentox.2008.07.013.

Wilhelmsen, Michael, Ib J. Christensen, Louise Rasmussen, Lars N. Jørgensen, Mogens R. Madsen, Jesper Vilandt, Thore Hillig, et al. 2017. "Detection of Colorectal Neoplasia: Combination of Eight Blood-

Based, Cancer-Associated Protein Biomarkers." *International Journal of Cancer* 140 (6): 1436–46. https://doi.org/10.1002/ijc.30558.

Williams, A. E. 2008. "Functional Aspects of Animal MicroRNAs." *Cellular and Molecular Life Sciences*. https://doi.org/10.1007/s00018-007-7355-9.

Wong, Thian Sze, Xiao Bing Liu, Birgitta Yee Hang Wong, Raymond Wai Man Ng, Anthony Po Wing Yuen, and William Ignace Wei. 2008. "Mature MiR-184 as Potential Oncogenic MicroRNA of Squamous Cell Carcinoma of Tongue." *Clinical Cancer Research* 14 (9): 2588–92. https://doi.org/10.1158/1078-0432.CCR-07-0666.

Wong, Yong Kie, Li Tsu Lee, and Chung Ji Liu. 2011. "Hypermethylation of MGMT and DAPK Gene Promoters Is Associated with Tumorigenesis and Metastasis in Oral Squamous Cell Carcinoma." *Journal of Dental Sciences* 6 (3): 158–64. https://doi.org/10.1016/j.jds.2011.05.006.

Wood NH, Khammissa R, Meyerov R, Lemmer J, Feller L. n.d. *Actinic Cheilitis: A Case Report and a Review of the Literature.*

World Health Organization. 2016. "WHO | Oral Health." *Who.*

Wu, T., E. Giovannucci, J. Welge, P. Mallick, W. Y. Tang, and S. M. Ho. 2011. "Measurement of GSTP1 Promoter Methylation in Body Fluids May Complement PSA Screening: A Meta-Analysis." *British Journal of Cancer* 105 (1): 65–73. https://doi.org/10.1038/bjc.2011.143.

Wu, Yanlin, Qiping Meng, Zhixue Yang, Lili Shi, Rongkuan Hu, Peizhuo Zhang, Jinrong Wei, et al. 2018. "Circulating HER-2 MRNA in the Peripheral Blood as a Potential Diagnostic and Prognostic Biomarker in Females with Breast Cancer." *Oncology Letters* 16 (3): 3726–34. https://doi.org/10.3892/ol.2018.9091.

Wu, Yansheng, Li Zhang, Lun Zhang, Yang Wang, Hui Li, Xiubao Ren, Feng Wei, et al. 2015. "Long Non-Coding RNA HOTAIR Promotes Tumor Cell Invasion and Metastasis by Recruiting EZH2 and Repressing E-Cadherin in Oral Squamous Cell Carcinoma." *International Journal of Oncology* 46 (6): 2586–94. https://doi.org/10.3892/ijo.2015.2976.

Xu, Huanxi, Yuqi Yang, Hongmei Zhao, Xuguang Yang, Yu Luo, Yinxiang Ren, Wei Liu, and Ning Li. 2016. "Serum MiR-483-5p: A Novel Diagnostic and Prognostic Biomarker for Patients with Oral Squamous Cell Carcinoma." *Tumor Biology* 37 (1): 447–53. https://doi.org/10.1007/s13277-015-3514-z.

Xu, Ran, Guang Zeng, Jing Gao, Yue Ren, Zhe Zhang, Qingna Zhang, Jinxiu Zhao, Hong Tao, and Daxu Li. 2015. "MIR-138 Suppresses the Proliferation of Oral Squamous Cell Carcinoma Cells by Targeting Yes-Associated Protein 1." *Oncology Reports* 34 (4): 2171–78. https://doi.org/10.3892/or.2015.4144.

Xue, Liying, Jinglong Nan, Li Dong, Cuiying Zhang, Hui Li, Rentuya Na, Huijie He, and Yadi Wang. 2017. "Upregulated MiR-483-5p Expression as a Prognostic Biomarker for Esophageal Squamous Cell Carcinoma." *Cancer Biomarkers* 19 (2): 193–97. https://doi.org/10.3233/CBM-160506.

Yamamoto, Hiroyuki, and Kohzoh Imai. 2015. "Microsatellite Instability: An Update." *Archives of Toxicology* 89 (6): 899–921. https://doi.org/10.1007/s00204-015-1474-0.

Yan, Yan, Xuan Wang, Morten T. Venø, Vivi Bakholdt, Jens A. Sørensen, Annelise Krogdahl, Zheng Sun, Shan Gao, and Jørgen Kjems. 2017. "Circulating MiRNAs as Biomarkers for Oral Squamous Cell Carcinoma Recurrence in Operated Patients." *Oncotarget* 8 (5): 8206–14. https://doi.org/10.18632/oncotarget.14143.

Yang, Bing, Zheng Liu, Hao Ning, Kai Zhang, Dongliang Pan, Kejia DIng, Wei Huang, Xin Li Kang, Yang Wang, and Xiang Chen. 2016. "MicroRNA-21 in Peripheral Blood Mononuclear Cells as a Novel Biomarker in the Diagnosis and Prognosis of Prostate Cancer." *Cancer Biomarkers* 17 (2): 223–30. https://doi.org/10.3233/CBM-160634.

Yang, Shih Wei, Yun Shien Lee, Liang Che Chang, Cheng Cheng Hwang, Cheng Ming Luo, and Tai An Chen. 2015. "Clinical Characteristics of Narrow-Band Imaging of Oral Erythroplakia and Its Correlation with Pathology." *BMC Cancer* 15 (1). https://doi.org/10.1186/s12885-015-1422-7.

Yang, Yan, Junwei Huang, Bahareh Rabii, Ramin Rabii, and Shen Hu. 2014. "Quantitative Proteomic Analysis of Serum Proteins from Oral Cancer Patients: Comparison of Two Analytical Methods." *International Journal of Molecular Sciences* 15 (8): 14386–95. https://doi.org/10.3390/ijms150814386.

Yang, Zhao Yang, Fang Yang, Ying Li Zhang, Bao Liu, Meng Wang, Xuan Hong, Yan Yu, Yao Hui Zhou, and Hai Zeng. 2017. "LncRNA-ANCR down-Regulation Suppresses Invasion and Migration of Colorectal Cancer Cells by Regulating EZH2 Expression." *Cancer Biomarkers* 18 (1): 95–104. https://doi.org/10.3233/CBM-161715.

Yang, Zongcheng, Xiuming Liang, Yue Fu, Yingjiao Liu, Lixin Zheng, Fen Liu, Tongyu Li, Xiaolin Yin, Xu Qiao, and Xin Xu. 2019. "Identification of AUNIP as a Candidate Diagnostic and Prognostic Biomarker for Oral Squamous Cell Carcinoma." *EBioMedicine* 47: 44–57. https://doi.org/10.1016/j.ebiom.2019.08.013.

Yao, Jin Guang, Lin Bo Gao, Yun Guang Liu, Jun Li, and Guang Fu Pang. 2008. "Genetic Variation in Interleukin-10 Gene and Risk of Oral Cancer." *Clinica Chimica Acta* 388 (1–2): 84–88. https://doi.org/10.1016/j.cca.2007.10.012.

Yao, Jun Tao, Shu Hong Zhao, Qiu Ping Liu, Mo Qi Lv, Dang Xia Zhou, Zi Jun Liao, and Ke Jun Nan. 2017. "Over-Expression of CircRNA_100876 in Non-Small Cell Lung Cancer and Its Prognostic Value." *Pathology Research and Practice* 213 (5): 453–56. https://doi.org/10.1016/j.prp.2017.02.011.

Yen, Yi Chen, Shine Gwo Shiah, Hsiao Chien Chu, Yuan Ming Hsu, Jenn Ren Hsiao, Jang Yang Chang, Wen Chun Hung, et al. 2014. "Reciprocal Regulation of MicroRNA-99a and Insulin-like Growth Factor I Receptor Signaling in Oral Squamous Cell Carcinoma Cells." *Molecular Cancer* 13 (1): 6. https://doi.org/10.1186/1476-4598-13-6.

Yoshimoto, Maisa, Jean Claude Cutz, Paulo A. S. Nuin, Anthony M. Joshua, Jane Bayani, Andrew J. Evans, Maria Zielenska, and Jeremy A. Squire. 2006. "Interphase FISH Analysis of PTEN in Histologic Sections Shows Genomic Deletions in 68% of Primary Prostate Cancer and 23% of High-Grade Prostatic Intra-Epithelial Neoplasias." *Cancer Genetics and*

Cytogenetics 169 (2): 128–37. https://doi.org/10.1016/j.cancergencyto.2006.04.003.

Yu, Lei, Xuejun Gong, Lei Sun, Qiying Zhou, Baoling Lu, and Liying Zhu. 2016. "The Circular RNA Cdr1as Act as an Oncogene in Hepatocellular Carcinoma through Targeting MiR-7 Expression." *PLoS ONE* 11 (7). https://doi.org/10.1371/journal.pone.0158347.

Zahran, F., D. Ghalwash, O. Shaker, K. Al-Johani, and C. Scully. 2015. "Salivary MicroRNAs in Oral Cancer." *Oral Diseases* 21 (6): 739–47. https://doi.org/10.1111/odi.12340.

Zamay, Tatiana, Galina Zamay, Olga Kolovskaya, Ruslan Zukov, Marina Petrova, Ana Gargaun, Maxim Berezovski, and Anna Kichkailo. 2017. "Current and Prospective Protein Biomarkers of Lung Cancer." *Cancers* 9 (12): 155. https://doi.org/10.3390/cancers9110155.

Zeng, Dequan, Hao Xu, Ning Ji, Jing Li, Min Zhou, Hongxia Dan, Yu Zhou, Xin Zeng, Lu Jiang, and Qianming Chen. 2019. "In Situ Measurement of MiR-138 Expression in Oral Squamous Cell Carcinoma Tissue Supports the Role of This MicroRNA as a Tumor Suppressor." *Journal of Oral Pathology and Medicine* 48 (10): 911–18. https://doi.org/10.1111/jop.12933.

Zeng, Guang, Wenxing Xun, Kewen Wei, Yongjin Yang, and Huan Shen. 2016. "MicroRNA-27a-3p Regulates Epithelial to Mesenchymal Transition via Targeting YAP1 in Oral Squamous Cell Carcinoma Cells." *Oncology Reports* 36 (3): 1475–82. https://doi.org/10.3892/or.2016.4916.

Zhang, Biru, Zihong Wang, Yuehong Shen, and Hongyu Yang. 2020. "Silencing Circular RNA Hsa_circ_009755 Promotes Growth and Metastasis of Oral Squamous Cell Carcinoma." *Genomics* 112 (6): 5275–81. https://doi.org/10.1016/j.ygeno.2020.09.035.

Zhao, Si-Yu, Jun Wang, Shao-Bo Ouyang, Zi-Kun Huang, and Lan Liao. 2018. "Salivary Circular RNAs Hsa_Circ_0001874 and Hsa_Circ_0001971 as Novel Biomarkers for the Diagnosis of Oral Squamous Cell Carcinoma." *Cellular Physiology and Biochemistry* 47 (6): 2511–21. https://doi.org/10.1159/000491624.

Zhao, Yanying, Qing Ren, and Kongxi Zhu. 2018. "Serum MiR-106b Upregulation Predicts Poor Prognosis in Patients with Colorectal Cancer." *International Journal of Clinical and Experimental Pathology* 11 (8): 4197–4204.

Zhou, Shan Shan, Jing Peng Jin, Ji Qun Wang, Zhi Guo Zhang, Jonathan H. Freedman, Yang Zheng, and Lu Cai. 2018. "MiRNAS in Cardiovascular Diseases: Potential Biomarkers, Therapeutic Targets and Challenges Review-Article." *Acta Pharmacologica Sinica.* Nature Publishing Group. https://doi.org/10.1038/aps.2018.30.

Zhou, Tao, and Yanjing Gao. 2016. "Increased Expression of LncRNA BANCR and Its Prognostic Significance in Human Hepatocellular Carcinoma." *World Journal of Surgical Oncology* 14 (1): 1–8. https://doi.org/10.1186/s12957-015-0757-5.

Zimmermann B. G., Wong D. T. n.d. "Salivary MRNA Targets for Cancer Diagnostics. *Oral Oncology.* 2008 May 1;44(5):425-9."

In: Oral Squamous Cell Carcinoma
Editor: Matthew Rabin
ISBN: 978-1-53619-895-9

Chapter 2

BUCCAL ORAL MUCOSAL DRUG DELIVERY SYSTEMS FOR TREATMENT AND ADJUVANT THERAPY OF ORAL CARCINOMA

Sabrina Barbosa de Souza Ferreira and Marcos Luciano Bruschi*
Postgraduate Program in Pharmaceutical Sciences,
Department of Pharmacy, State University of Maringa,
Maringa, PR, Brazil

ABSTRACT

Oral squamous cell carcinoma is the third most common type of malignancy in developing countries and the eighth most common in developed countries. The rate survival is poor when there is late detection of these lesions. The development of oral mucosal drug delivery systems may be quite useful as treatment and as adjuvant of oral cancer. This chapter is focused on principles, systems, technology, therapeutic approaches, safety and toxicity and patents comprising drug delivery systems for local oral squamous cell carcinoma treatment. In this context,

* Corresponding Author's E-mail: mlbruschi@uem.br.

the most valuable and up-to-date oral drug delivery systems for oral squamous cell carcinoma were discussed. Some aspects and definitions were revised in terms of oral mucosal environment, challenges, and benefits of local treatment of oral squamous cell carcinoma, as well as the characteristics of the active pharmaceutical ingredients. The strategies to foster the drug delivery, the advances in both *in vitro* and *in vivo* activity, and patents and registered products in the market aiming local treatment of oral squamous cell carcinoma were considered.

Keywords: oral, OSCC, drug delivery, treatment, therapy.

Introduction

Oral squamous cell carcinoma (OSCC) represents 91% of all head and neck malignancies, and it has been considered a challenge for head and neck surgeons (Hsu et al. 2014; Narihira et al. 2018; Gatta et al. 2015; Capote-Moreno et al. 2020). OSCC is the eightieth the most common malignancy in developed countries and the third most common type of cancer in developing countries (Srivastava et al. 2018).

New therapeutic options emerged for OSCC and metastatic OSCC during the last decades, including chemotherapy, radiotherapy, immunotherapy, surgical procedures, photodynamic therapy and photothermal therapy. The surgical modalities have provided better aesthetic results with improved quality of life for patients due to larger surgical resections and primary reconstruction of defects. New radiation and chemotherapy modalities try to improve survival. Moreover, immunotherapy has been introduced to improve the immune system against the tumoral cells (Ghanizada et al. 2019; Samra et al. 2018; Ding et al. 2020). Despite the advances in surgical techniques and new therapies, recent studies have demonstrated that the recurrence and survival rates (50-60%) have not improved keeping around 2-3 years (Capote-Moreno et al. 2020; Tiwana et al. 2014).

The use of strategies to modify the drug release and enable the availability of the active pharmaceutical ingredients with improved safety and efficacy by controlling the rate, time and site of drug release are called drug delivery systems (Ferreira and Bruschi 2019; Bruschi 2015). Over the last three decades, researchers have developed buccal drug delivery systems with enhanced therapeutic efficacy of ineffective drugs carried by traditional pharmaceutical dosage forms (Meher et al. 2013; Gowthamarajan et al. 2012).

However, this administration route is considered a challenge to the pharmaceutical industry and scientists due to the complexity of oral cavity. The comprehension of oral cavity anatomy and physiology, including salivary flow, the keratinization pattern in different regions of oral cavity and permeability may influence in the drug delivery performance (Meher et al. 2013; Gowthamarajan et al. 2012). In addition, it is quite important to understand the components of pharmaceutical dosage form to achieve the optimized therapy (Taylor and Aulton 2017).

It is quite known that the physiopathology of OSCC may change the characteristics and physiology of the oral mucosa. The knowledge of these alterations, including pH, salivary flow and permeation show huge importance for the development of drug delivery systems which aims the OSCC treatment (Colley et al. 2014; Ferreira et al. 2020). Nanotechnology and other pharmaceutical dosage forms represent new therapeutic options to improve the survival and life quality of patients affected with OSCC (Ding et al. 2020; Chandran et al. 2011; Hafizi et al. 2019). In addition, this therapeutic approach could be used as a local treatment and as adjuvant for the therapy.

This chapter is focused on describing definitions, systems, technology, and advances in oral mucosal drug delivery systems for the treatment and adjuvant therapy of OSCC. The fundamentals in terms of oral mucosal environment in oral cancer, the challenges, and benefits of OSCC local treatment, and the physicochemical characteristics of active pharmaceutical ingredients are revised. The strategies to modify drug release, technology, and pharmaceutical forms are discussed. The safety and toxicity of these formulations are also addressed. In addition, the patents and market are also considered.

DEFINITIONS AND FUNDAMENTALS

Oral Mucosal Environment in Oral Cancer as a Route for Drug Administration

The oral cavity, especially oral mucosa, is a promising route for drug delivery in oral cancer. This is a complex environment, and the knowledge of the histology, physiology and pathophysiology of this region displays huge importance in the development of optimized formulations (Bruschi, Ferreira, and Silva 2020). The main factors which could interfere in the performance of drug delivery systems would be the location in oral cavity, the thickness and keratinization pattern of oral mucosa and salivary flow, pH (5.5-7.0) and composition (Bruschi and de Freitas 2005; Bruschi, Ferreira, and Silva 2020; Patel, Liu, and Brown 2012; Palem et al. 2013; Sandri et al. 2020). These characteristics may change during development and the stage of OSCC, and it should also be understood during the development of drug delivery systems for the oral cancer treatment.

The permeability of drugs may be affected by the stratification and keratinization pattern of oral mucosa, that may be keratinized and non-keratinized (Bruschi and de Freitas 2005; Patel, Liu, and Brown 2012). The keratinized epithelium covers the masticatory mucosa in the structures of gum and hard palate areas. The neutral lipids, including ceramides and acylceramides, which are found in keratinized epithelium, are responsible for the lower permeability to water. While few polar lipids (cholesterol sulphate and glucosylceramides) are found in non-keratinized epithelium (Smart 1993; Sudhakar, Kuotsu, and Bandyopadhyay 2006; Morantes et al. 2017; Russo et al. 2016). This type of epithelium covers the lining mucosa in buccal and labial mucosa, ventral tongue, soft palate and vestibular and floor of mouth (Sudhakar, Kuotsu, and Bandyopadhyay 2006; Morantes et al. 2017; Teubl et al. 2013; Mortazavi and Smart 1993). In addition, the presence of lipid membrane coating granules is the major predictor of permeability of the buccal mucosa and is involved in the formation of a protective layer over the oral mucosa (Said 2018; Salamat-Miller, Chittchang, and Johnston 2005).

In physiological conditions, the location of drug administration may interfere in its permeability due to the combination of thickness and keratinization pattern of oral mucosa. For example, the administration of drugs in gingival and hard palate mucosae (keratinized epithelium) may be useful for local delivery of drugs and treat localized diseases, including oral cancer. Sublingual mucosa is thinner, highly vascularized, and consequently, useful for systemic administration of drugs with fast activity in acute disorders (e.g., angina pectoris). Cheek or buccal mucosa, which is less permeable than the sublingual mucosa, is suitable for prolonged therapies due to the relative immobile surface, for both local and systemic disorders. In addition, this is more permeable than other oral cavity regions (except sublingual mucosa) (Sandri et al. 2020; Palem et al. 2013).

Besides the performance of the drug delivery system, the keratinization pattern is also considered as a histopathological parameter for OSCC development (Dissanayaka et al. 2012). According to the gene involved in the development of OSCC, it has been observed a specific survival rate and keratinization pattern. This relation may also interfere in the development of drug delivery systems with specific characteristics. Undifferentiated tissues have shown lower keratinization patterns and are related with lower survival rates of OSCC patients, in comparison to keratinized tissues display higher survival rate (Pinto et al. 2010).

The aspects related to the saliva, including flow, composition and pH can also interfere in the performance and desirable characteristics of drug delivery systems. These aspects may change in physiological and pathological conditions. Saliva displays a range of homeostatic and physiological functions, including a contribution to initial digestion and formation of bolus and remineralization of enamel. In normal conditions, it is produced 0.5-2.0 L of saliva per day, with flow rate near 0.5 mL/min. The major composition in saliva is water (99.5%) followed by solutes (0.5%), such as ions, enzymes, proteins, and organic compounds. The flow and composition are variable according to the stimulus (basal or stimulated) (Bruschi and de Freitas 2005; Smart 1993; Nagai and Machida 1993; Sudhakar, Kuotsu, and Bandyopadhyay 2006; Chiappin et al. 2007).

Besides the changes in salivary flow and viscosity in pathological conditions, the radiotherapy treatment have been reported to cause hyposalivation and xerostomia, with consequent tooth decay, periodontal disease, and dysphagia and thick salivary secretions (Bomeli et al. 2008; Kaae, Stenfeldt, and Eriksen 2016). Lalla and co-authors (2017) have reported the decrease in stimulated salivary flow rate from 1.09 mL/min to 0.47 mL/min after six months from the beginning of radiotherapy in a cohort study (Lalla et al. 2017). The opposite condition has been also reported as a less frequent complication (Bomeli et al. 2008) by the excess of salivary flow or sialorrhea due to the tumor location or treatment related dysphagia. Some chemotherapeutic drugs may change the salivary flow, viscosity and its composition interfering in the amount of lysozyme, lactoperoxidases, lactoferrins which has antimicrobial activity (Pereira et al. 2015).

During the development of drug delivery systems for OSCC, it is important that they can adapt to these conditions and keep the therapeutic efficacy.

Challenges and Benefits of the Local Treatment of OSCC

Considering the oral cancer traditional chemotherapy treatment, the most common administration route is intravenous due to improved absorption and bioavailability. However, there are some drawbacks, including increased risk of side effects (nausea, vomiting, hair loss, infections, and diarrhea) and the possibility to affect normal tissues (Sledge and Miller 2003; Ding et al. 2020; Ketabat et al. 2019).

Over the last decades, researchers have studied the development of local drug delivery systems (controlled and/or prolonged release) as alternative therapeutic approaches to provide benefits for current anticancer therapies (Bruschi 2015; Ketabat et al. 2019). These formulations promote the uniform release, decrease the number and frequency of doses required to the therapeutic effect and decrease the side effects, increasing the adhesion of the patient to the therapy (Carvalho et al. 2010; Nho, Park, and Lim 2014).

However, it is necessary to pay attention to its benefits and challenges to achieve the therapeutic effect.

Among the benefits of local treatment of OSCC, the conveniency, facilitated prolonged exposure to the anticancer drugs (Anaya et al. 2019; Ding et al. 2020), minimized undesirable toxic effects on healthy cells and patient compliance have been reported in literature (Ketabat et al. 2019; Calixto et al. 2014). These formulations may release the drug at a specific location with a specific delivery rate. Besides, enhanced drug availability and biodistribution at the site of tumor have been described by these targeted drug delivery systems. Some authors have also discussed the potential for outpatient treatment by enhancing the drug efficiency while reducing the treatment period with lower healthcare expenses (Ketabat et al. 2019; O'neill and Twelves 2002). Targeted drug delivery systems may also improve the half-time of easy degradable bioactive molecules (proteins and peptides) and prolong their local effects, as demonstrated by *in vivo* studies (O'neill and Twelves 2002; Ketabat et al. 2019).

The biological environment, as previously discussed, represents a challenge in the development of buccal drug delivery systems due to the possible impairment of therapeutic efficacy. The formulation may suffer salivary dilution and dissolution and the possible swallowing of the drug delivery systems leading to suffocation (Russo et al. 2016; Sudhakar, Kuotsu, and Bandyopadhyay 2006; Salamat-Miller, Chittchang, and Johnston 2005; Morantes et al. 2017; Patel, Liu, and Brown 2012). It is also important that the targeted drug delivery system should be developed according to the disease stage and be able to permeate according to the keratinization pattern. Low solubility in aqueous solutions, low apparent permeation and poor bioavailability may represent a limitation and challenge of oral route administration (Calixto et al. 2014; Devalapally, Chakilam, and Amiji 2006; Agüeros et al. 2009; Anaya et al. 2019; Ding et al. 2020).

Suitable Physicochemical and Biopharmaceuticals Characteristics of the Active Pharmaceutical Ingredients

Some physicochemical properties such as solubility, partition coefficient, ionization degree and molecular weight of the active pharmaceutical ingredients may influence the performance of oral mucosal drug delivery systems (Satheesh Madhav et al. 2012). The main aspects which suffer this influence are the permeability, availability, and distribution for cancer cells. The potency of the active pharmaceutical ingredient is also quite important and desirable by using low quantities to achieve the suitable oral activity over cancer cells (Zhang H., Zhang J., and Streisand J. B. 2002). Some authors reported that anticancer agents have diverse limitations regarding oral bioavailability, stability in natural conditions and non-specific biodistribution by influencing the therapeutic efficacy (Ketabat et al. 2019; Pérez-Herrero and Fernández-Medarde 2015; Masood 2016).

The solubility and the partition coefficient of active pharmaceutical ingredient impact directly in the permeability and it is necessary to have a balance between these two characteristics to be administered by oral mucosal route (Fonseca-Santos and Chorilli 2018; Zhang H., Zhang J., and Streisand J. B. 2002). Drugs with hydrophilic nature tend to permeate by paracellular pathway (around and between the cells) and hydrophobic drugs are preferably absorbed by transcellular route (Sangeetha et al. 2010; Morantes et al. 2017; Satheesh Madhav et al. 2012; Patel, Liu, and Brown 2012). The last ones may cross the lipophilic cell membrane by carrier-mediated transport, pinocytosis, and transmembrane passive diffusion. Inside the cell, these drugs can form a vesicle which crosses the other side of the opposite cell side (Sangeetha et al. 2010; Sagiri et al. 2015; Patel, Liu, and Brown 2012; Y. Guo and Pratap Singh 2019). Increased partition coefficient due to intramolecular hydrogen bonds may increase the permeability of hydrophilic drugs in physiological environments (pH ~6 – 6.6) (Y. Guo and Pratap Singh 2019; Morales and McConville 2014).

The permeability of active pharmaceutical ingredients may be affected by its molecular weight and size. Molecules showing high molecular weight (from 600 Da to 100 kDa) display complex and low permeability in comparison to small structures (<100 Da) which may permeate the oral mucosa easily (Morales and McConville 2014). In addition, the ionizable hydrophilic drugs also may affect its permeability, like proteins and peptides. The non-ionizable state favors the transcellular route of permeation. Ionized state of drugs encourages paracellular pathway of permeability (Y. Guo and Pratap Singh 2019; Puratchikody et al. 2011).

DRUG DELIVERY SYSTEMS FOR LOCAL TREATMENT OF ORAL SQUAMOUS CELL CARCINOMA

Considering the limitations of radiotherapy and surgery, the utilization of chemotherapy in OSCC continues to improve and also driven due to the low sensitivity of oral cancer cells to antineoplastic active agents. OSCC is most common for both genders worldwide and oral sites such as tongue, sublingual region, cheek, pharynx, and palates (hard and soft) are mainly committed. As previously described, these regions have particular characteristics as pH, humidity, salivary flow presence, mucin presence, mechanical movements (like during the speaking and chewing), and sometimes presence of food as well.

The development of novel methodologies and technologies to eradicate OSCC cells with minimal adverse effects on normal cells is very important. In other words, the drug delivery systems should enable an effective, selective and safety therapy. During the treatment of OSCC (prevention, adjuvant therapy and therapy), it is also necessary to consider that the patient can be under different protocols based on tumor stage, such as chemoradiation and induction chemotherapy. Therefore, some anticancer agents have been used alone or in combination, such as doxorubicin, cetuximab, fluoropyrimidine 5-fluorouracil, cisplatin, bleomycin, docetaxel, paclitaxel, methotrexate, ellagic acid, and compounds from natural sources such as curcumin, propolis, genistein, black raspberry (Hulpuch et al. 2010; Ding et al. 2020; Ketabat et al. 2019; Ferreira et al. 2020; Esposito et al. 2020; Bonner et al. 2010; Adelstein et al. 2003; Scully and Bagan 2009).

Moreover, monoclonal antibodies have also been utilized (Ketabat et al. 2019).

The oral buccal administration may display environments quite or totally different from the physiological. They are particular environments, and it is also important to consider that OSCC is a malignant tumor showing rapid spreading on the most of the cases.

Therefore, the use of strategies for modification of drug delivery can improve the local therapy of OSCC tumors, increasing the safety, effectiveness, and quality of the treatment. Moreover, the controlled drug delivery can reduce side effects. In this context, new technologies and innovative systems have been proposed for the local administration of anticancer drugs for OSCC aiming the prevention and the therapy.

Strategies

Parenteral administration of anticancer agents, mainly intravenous route, is the most direct and can overcome some barriers and variables that can limit the drug bioavailability, like the variations of absorption patterns when the drug is administered through the gastrointestinal tract.

Intravenous route can enable the immediate and complete bioavailability of the anticancer agent; however, this administration route can deliver high drug concentrations to normal tissues, causing adverse effects and damage to healthy tissues as well.

In addition, some drugs show the ability for reach the blood circulation fatly by the blood capillary wall. Colloids can be drained by the lymphatic system at the same time, and these routes of administration (intratumor and peritumoral injections) are regarded as a tool for lymphatic targeting and are the predominant administration methods for the treatment of oral cancer, mainly in the field of photodynamic therapy (PDT) and photothermal therapy (PTT) (Ding et al. 2020). However, it is necessary to consider that these routes are highly invasive and not comfortable for the patient (Rathbone, 1996).

Therefore, besides the improved safety, the convenience and potential for outpatient treatment lead the oral buccal administration of anticancer drugs to be preferred by patients with OSCC. The local administration can improve the prolonged exposure to an anticancer agent, and the oral mucosal route of administration shows the potential to improve the local effects while reducing systemic undesirable effects.

Novel drug delivery systems for oral mucosal administration have the aim to release the drug within a defined and suitable period. However, it is necessary to consider the physicochemical characteristics of the active agent such as solubility and permeability. They can conduce for a high or poor drug bioavailability and may be limitations for the oral chemotherapy (Bruschi and de Freitas 2005; Agüeros et al. 2009; Calixto et al. 2014).

It is necessary that the system displays a high drug loading capacity, easiness of administration with no or minimal discomfort to the patient, improved retention time at the site of administration, non-irritancy, good feel in the oral cavity, tastelessness, and controlled delivery of the active agent. In most of the cases, it is desirable that the formulation displays biodegradability or easy removal after the total drug release.

Technology

Many types of oral mucosal dosage forms have been suggested, such as solid systems (e.g., tablets, patches and particulate systems) and semisolid systems (e.g., gels and emulsion systems). In addition, the use of polymeric materials and nanotechnology for the development of drug delivery systems for OSCC treatment has been described mainly during the last decade to overcome disadvantages of the current protocols and techniques utilized for the OSCC treatment (Calixto et al. 2014).

Nanotechnology can collaborate for the improvement of the efficacy of the chemotherapeutic regimens, which is closely related to targeting the oral cancer cells and avoiding the damage of normal cells as minimal as possible. Moreover, the nanotechnology can also contribute for detection of occult tumors or precancerous lesions, making them more visible through image examinations (Ding et al. 2020). This technology showed to be valid for targeting cancer cells and produce less cytotoxic effects on normal tissues. Many investigations have displayed important results relating the new nanotechnological therapeutic options to the improvement of the survival time and the quality life of the cancer patients (Calixto et al. 2014; Ding et al. 2020).

The phenomenon of attachment between two surfaces is defined as adhesion. The adhesion processes are an important strategy to be used in diverse healthcare and non-biomedical implications (Mathiowitz et al. 1999). The process of a pharmaceutical system to come into close contact with the mucosal surface is called mucoadhesion (Andrews, Laverty, and Jones 2009; Mansuri et al. 2016; Bruschi and de Freitas 2005; Ferreira et al. 2015; Khutoryanskiy 2011; Cook and Khutoryanskiy 2015; da Silva et al. 2018; da Silva et al. 2017). Mucoadhesive systems can provide intimate contact between the mucosal tissue and the dosage form, which can improved the drug amount in a specific area and therefore, increase the drug flux through the absorbing tissue and improved drug availability (Rathbone, 1996; Mathiowitz et al. 1999; Bruschi and de Freitas 2005).

Environmentally responsive materials (e.g., polymers) can help the development of pharmaceutical systems with the capacity to change their physical properties, such as shape, permeability, solubility, physical state as well as mechanical, optical, and electrical properties, upon environmental conditions vary. Moreover, once the external trigger is removed, they can return to their original properties as well (Bruschi, Borghi-Pangoni, Junqueira, and Ferreira 2017).

The types of stimulus that can promote structural changes in responsive systems may be classified in three main groups: physical (e.g., temperature, ultrasound, light, electric field or mechanical stress), chemical (e.g., pH and ionic strength) and biological (e.g., enzymes) (Almeida et al. 2013). The most reported stimuli are pH, temperature, ionic strength, and light (Bruschi, Borghi-Pangoni, Junqueira, and Ferreira 2017).

Temperature-responsive systems can display high versatility in design, tenability of phase transition temperatures, passive targeting ability and in situ phase transitions (Bikram and West, 2008). Their physical properties can alter due to temperature changes, and the sol-gel transition can occur due to the properties of polymers. At a determined temperature, a volume phase transition of polymers can cause an abrupt alteration in the solvation state. These phenomena or the variation of the hydration state can be related to the intra and/or intermolecular attractive forces of the polymers' chains that are more favorable than solubilization by water. The balance of hydrophilic and hydrophobic groups can govern the abrupt change the solubility as a little temperature change. Many synthetic and naturally-occurring polymers can show these characteristics, such as chitosan, cellulose, gelatin, xyloglucan, poly(ethylene oxide)-b-poly(propylene oxide)-b-poly(ethylene oxide) (PEO/PPO/PEO) block copolymers, poly-N-isopropylacrylamide (pNiPAAm), poly(ethylene oxide)–b–poly(D,L-lactic acid co-glycolic acid)-b-poly(ethylene oxide) (PEO/PLGA/PEO) triblock copolymers, and amphiphilic triblock copolymers, composed of poly-caprolactone (PCL) and PEO (PEO/PCL/PEO) (Ruel-Gariépy 2004; Bruschi, Borghi-Pangoni, Junqueira, and Ferreira 2017).

Another strategy is to use pH responsive/sensitive polymers for drug delivery systems to be applied at the oral mucosa. These materials respond to small pH changes in the environment and their solubility, conformation, hydrophilic/hydrophobic balance alteration or the release of a bioactive agent can alter as well. A polymer showing pKa value between 3 and 10 and is ionizable seems to be candidate to compose pH-responsive systems. For example, weak bases and acids like amines, phosphoric acid, and carboxylic acids, display a change in the ionization state in response to pH variation, resulting in a conformational change in the swelling behavior of the polymeric matrix, when these ionizable groups are connected to the polymer structure (Schmaljohann et al. 2006). Therefore, it is possible to modulate the active agent delivery at a specific pH response local on the mucosa.

Light responsive materials are also extremely attractive, since they display some important advantages in relationship to pH and temperature, such as easy-to-manipulate and externally induced with precise spatial and temporal control. Moreover, it is possible to use materials that are responsive to innocuous radiation (Alvarez-Lorenzo et al. 2009; Yang et al. 2016). In addition, modern laser systems allow a precise control of light intensity, duration, wavelength, and the diameter of the beam offer a broad range of possibilities for biomedical applications. For example, UV or blue light, ranges from 15 a 490 nm, is commonly applied for local treatments to mucosa (Bruschi, Borghi-Pangoni, Junqueira, Ferreira, et al. 2017). UV radiation (190 – 400 nm) cannot penetrate more than 1 cm into the tissue, which can limit the treatment of pathological processes. However, systems activated by near-infrared irradiation of UV (650 to 900 nm) emitting up converting nanoparticles have been proposed for the increase of penetration in the tissue (Fong et al. 2016). Thus, this strategy may be useful in precisely controlled release of active agents intended for difficult access areas of the mouth and for direct photothermal killing of cancer cells (Alvarez-Lorenzo et al. 2009). Systems composed of light-responsive materials have been developed for a single use, due the irreversible structural change triggered by light that results the delivery of the entire dose.

Pharmaceutical systems for oral mucosal administration composed of these smart materials are biocompatible, biodegradable and can also display improved drug delivery efficiency and accuracy. They can lead the active agent to the target cells and release in a triggered way. These formulations can sometimes mimic the physiological homeostatic feedback mechanisms which are essential for health (Siegel, 2014). Moreover, these systems should be eliminated after performing their aim. However, depending upon the composition and the target tissue, they can be withdrawn using stool or if necessary, to tailor their degradability in organism (Bruschi and de Freitas 2005; Bruschi, Borghi-Pangoni, Junqueira, and Ferreira 2017).

Some types of light are utilized since the ancient times as phototherapy of many topical disorders, such as the sunlight. In this context, the photodynamic therapy (PDT) includes irradiation therapy, phototherapy or photochemotherapy, which constitutes a good option for the treatment of several types of diseases, including cancer (Boiy et al. 2011). PDT is a therapy that combines the administration of a photosensitizer agent followed by the irradiation of visible light for generation of reactive oxygen species (ROS), mainly singlet oxygen ($^1O_2$), which lead to the cytotoxic effects. Photosensitizer utilized in PDT can be from synthetic or natural origin, and methylene blue, hypericin, erythrosine-B, 5-aminolevulinic acid, and porphyrin derivatives are examples utilized for cancer PDT. The selectivity, activity and photophysical properties are important characteristics for a photosensitizer. Nowadays, there is an interest for the development of photosensitizers that show additional targeting mechanism, such as the capacity to attach to monoclonal antibodies (Choudhary et al. 2009; Bruschi et al. 2019).

Moreover, photo-thermal therapy (PTT) also employs light absorbing agents for generation of heat, which can damage cancer cells, reducing and eliminating the tumor. However, PTT can also damage the surrounding normal tissue due to the high laser density, which can difficult the clinical applications (Ketabat et al. 2019; R. Guo et al. 2016).

Sometimes, due to the physicochemical characteristics of the active agent, like solubility, and the necessity to improve the drug absorption, it is necessary to develop emulsion systems to carry it. Thus, the emulsifying process is a very suitable technological strategy to produce efficient platforms for oral mucosal drug delivery (Bruschi and de Freitas 2005). Emulsion hydrogels or emulgels are semi-solid systems composed by two phases, an inner insoluble and hydrophobic phase dispersed and in an external hydrophilic and continuous phase. These systems can be applied on the mucosa and can increase the residence time at the site of the administration. Emulgels can be prepared by the combination of the characteristics of oil/water or water/oil-emulsion and gel, which can result in suitable and effective release for both hydrophobic and hydrophilic active agents (Khullar et al. 2012; Burki et al. 2020). Emulgels are emulsions which have the dispersing (continuous) phase gelled by adding a gelling agent or an aqueous phase thickener. This gelling capacity conduces to the formation of emulsions with higher physicochemical stability due to the reduction of the interfacial tension and increasing the aqueous phase viscosity.

The use of phases of different polarities and surfactants can also lead to obtain liquid crystalline or mesomorphic phases. Liquid crystalline systems can be adhesive semi-solid systems improving their retention on the site of administration (Bruschi and de Freitas 2005; Bruschi et al. 2008; Calixto et al. 2014). Moreover, their improved mechanical and rheological characteristics, as well as the capacity to control de drug release, are suitable characteristics for their oral mucosal administration on the treatment of OSCC.

The use of magnetic nanoparticles, such as iron-oxide nanoparticles, has attracted great interest in pharmaceutical applications such as hyperthermia and drug delivery. Iron-oxide magnetic nanoparticles are chemically and physically stable, biocompatible, and environmentally safe. They can be designed to be stimulus responsive, and a magnetic field can stimulate the nanostructures that can act as an anticancer agent. The superparamagnetism, size, and the possibility of receiving a biocompatible coating enable these nanostructures for pharmaceutical applications in OSCC treatment (Bruschi and Toledo et al., 2019).

Mucoadhesive polymers (e.g., carbomers, others acrylic acid and cellulose derivatives) are particularly interesting for production of emulgel systems with mucoadhesive property. Therefore, emulgels can be used for controlled release of anticancer agents and to improve their availability in the tumor (Ferreira and Bruschi 2021). Moreover, the strategy to combine environmentally responsive and mucoadhesive materials have demonstrated many advantages, such as produce systems for reducing of dose frequency, with ease of preparation and administration, prolonged release, reduced side effects, and finally have reduced costs (Bruschi, Borghi-Pangoni, Junqueira, and Ferreira 2017).

The use of membranous vesicles displaying sizes between 40–120 nm has been also proposed for the treatment of OSCC (Ketabat et al. 2019). These structures are called exosomes and they can be secreted by macrophages, dendritic cells, mesenchymal stem cells, endothelial, and epithelial cells, into the extracellular space (Jiang and Gao 2017). They are secreted when the multivesicular body fuses with the plasma membrane, can carry different types of biomolecules, and play an essential role in intercellular communication, making them suitable carrier systems (Bunggulawa et al. 2018).

Exosomes have been investigated for delivery doxorubicin, curcumin, and paclitaxel, displaying reduction of their side effects and improved therapeutic efficiency (Sun et al. 2010; Tian et al. 2014; Batrakova and Kim 2015).

However, exosomes show some disadvantages, such as the limited capacity to deliver high amounts of therapeutic agents, their purification is a long and demanding process that usually generate low yields, and their administration might lead to adverse immune reactions (Ha et al., 2016). Therefore, the use of exosomes for the OSCC treatment is an important strategy, but their analysis, purification, and administration are still challenging (Luan et al. 2017; Ketabat et al. 2019).

Pharmaceutical Dosage Forms

A high number of pharmaceutical systems for buccal mucosal administration have been proposed and they are composed of different biomaterials, inorganic materials, and small molecules, aiming the optimization of the local/buccal treatment route (Calixto et al. 2014; Ding et al. 2020):

- Polymeric nanoparticles;
- Lipid systems (solid lipid nanoparticles and lipid nanocarriers);
- Liposomes;
- Cyclodextrin complex;
- Inorganic nanoparticles;
- Hydrogels;
- Emulgels;
- Liquid crystals.

However, as final dosage forms for oral mucosal administration, they can also be grouped into bioadhesive systems and chewing gums (Chidambaram and Srivatsava 1995; Bruschi and de Freitas 2005). Therefore, the following pharmaceutical systems have mainly been utilized as systems for delivery of active agents in the OSCC treatment: hydrogels, emulgels, polymeric nanoparticles, solid lipid nanoparticles, nanostructured lipid carriers, magnetic, nanoparticles, gold nanoparticles, cyclodextrin complexes, and liquid crystals.

As previously described, the use of strategies such as nanotechnology, bioadhesion and response to the environmental conditions can lead to the development of improved drug delivery systems, which can represent a particularly important option for the treatment of OSCC.

The use of natural, semi-synthetic and/or synthetic polymers to produce hydrogels for oral mucosal administration is an especially important strategy. Hydrogels are defined as three-dimensional polymer networks, with different degrees of cross-linking, and showing the ability to imbibe and retain large amount of water (Wang et al. 2020). Because of their tunable properties as well as their versatile fabrication methods, hydrogel materials have been used in a wide range of biomedical and pharmaceutical applications (Peppas et al. 2012; Wang et al. 2020).

Depending on the chain entanglements and chemical or physical cross-links, hydrogels cannot typically dissolve. Due to these characteristics, hydrogels can be used as platforms for modified and/or controlled drug release. They can constitute platforms for release bioactive agents for dissolution and disintegration through the spaces in their matrices.

The mechanical, rheological and bioadhesive properties of hydrogels can be modulated according to their chemical composition and structural characteristics. Therefore, these platforms are incredibly attractive for oral mucosal administration enabling the intimated contact with the tissue. Many anticancer agents are utilized alone or in combination for the current chemotherapy of OSCC, such as doxorubicin, tamoxifen, cisplatin, docetaxel, and paclitaxel have been investigated for administration using this kind of system composed of different polymers. Moreover, they can be used for the preparation of emulgels, which constitute a particularly important strategy, as previously described.

Lipid systems have been also proposed as drug delivery systems for oral mucosal treatment of OSCC (Calixto et al. 2014). Solid lipid nanoparticles have been considered one of the most impressive colloidal systems proposed on the last decades (Freitas and Müller 1998; Paranjipe et al. 2014; Rosseto et al. 2017).

These nanostructures can show physical stability, protection of active agents from degradation, controlled release, and excellent tolerability, which enabled their administration for different routes, such as oral (Freitas and Müller, 1998; Holpuch et al. 2010; Paranjipe et al. 2014).

They are prepared using solid lipids (at room temperature), surfactant and a dispersion technique, such as high-pressure homogenization (HPH) process or other methods that use organic solvents (HPH/solvent evaporation), or the dilution of microemulsions (Freitas and Müller, 1998; Rosseto et al. 2017).

In addition, nanostructured lipid carriers are prepared using a mixture of solid and liquid lipids (Krasodomska et al. 2016). They have emerged as a new generation of nanostructured lipid systems to avoid the drug degradation, the coexistence of different lipid modifications and colloidal species, and a low drug-loading capacity of some solid lipid nanoparticles prepared by use of the HPH process (Krasodomska et al. 2016; Rosseto et al. 2017).

The liquid lipid presence can form nanocompartments that avoid the solid lipid crystallization and enable the increase of the drug payload and improved drug release, because they are still controlled by a surrounding solid lipid barrier (Fang et al., 2008; Kovacevic et al., 2011). Lipid systems have been proposed for delivery of different anticancer agents (e.g., narigenin, ganciclovir, chlorin, idarubicin hydrochloride, curcumin, genistein, retinoic acid, docetaxel, etoposide, quercetin, and etoposide) as solid nanoparticles or nanostructured carriers.

For oral mucosal administration, these lipid systems can also be incorporated in a final dosage form with improve mucoadhesive characteristics. Studies have been proposed for the development of these new platforms, such as environmentally responsive, mucoadhesive and emulsion semi-solid systems (Holpuch et al. 2010; Ferreira et al. 2019; Ferreira et al. 2020).

In this context, liposomes have also been investigated as pharmaceutical systems for the treatment of OSCC. Different anticancer agents have been entrapped in liposomes, such as the photosensitizer aluminium phthalocyanine chloride, to be utilized in photodynamic therapy (Longo, Lozzi, and Azevedo 2011; Velloso et al. 2012). Despite liposomes are mainly utilized as drug delivery systems for the systemic administration for the treatment of OSCC, they can also be locally administered on the oral mucosal site using suitable platforms aiming the liposome protection and the increase of their accumulation at target site (Calixto et al. 2014).

The anticancer agents can be entrapped, solubilized, or attached to polymeric nanoparticles (Brannon-Peppas and Blanchette 2010; Holpuch et al. 2010; Chu et al. 2013). These supramolecular solid structures can act as matrix or reservoir systems for controlled delivery of anticancer agents (Mohanraj et al. 2006; Brewer et al. 2011; Makadia et al. 2011). They can be produced using different types of substances like biocompatible/ biodegradable polymers, polysaccharides and proteins. Nanoparticles composed of poly(D,L-lactide), poly(lactic acid) (PLA), poly(D,L-glycolide), poly(lactide-co-glycolide), polycyanoacrylate, polyethylene glycol (PEG), poly(γ-benzyl l-glutamate) (PBLG), gelatin, sodium alginate and chitosan. Thus, they have the advantage to be biodegradable, biocompatible and can show suitability for controlled and sustained release of active agents, improving the efficacy and reducing the side effects.

These nanoparticles are mainly produced using the dispersion of preformed polymers and other compounds, the polymerization of monomers, ionic gelation, coacervation of hydrophilic polymers, supercritical fluid technology and particle replication in non-wetting templates as well (Petros et al. 2010, Z. Wang et al. 2010; Fan et al. 2012; Dhanda et al. 2013; Calixto et al. 2014). They can improve the stability and control the targeted delivery of anticancer agents. In addition, polymeric nanoparticles can display mucoadhesive property and improve the retention time of system at the site of administration.

These characteristics are useful for allowing for a constant and uniform drug amount at the injured/ill tissue, enabling high concentration of active agent into the tumor, and the reduction of side effects as well (Calixto et al. 2014; Yu et al. 2009). Despite the incredibly attractive advantages, such as difficult to handle due to the particle-particle aggregation, not suitable for the release of proteins, and also problems of toxicity after cell internalization (Calixto et al. 2014; Ketabat et al. 2019), which can restrict their use, and this problem should be always considered during the development process of these nanocarriers.

Liquid crystals may be classified in thermotropics or lyotropics, which are structured by means of temperature or by association with amphipathic compounds and solvents, respectively. They are usually based on water as a solvent, surfactant (may contain cosurfactants), and an oily phase. Their physicochemical stability, mechanical and rheological characteristics, and the capacity to carry different types of anticancer agents make them important systems for oral mucosal administration. The liquid crystalline systems can control the release profile and reduce the toxicity of active agent, improving clinical efficiency (Calixto et al. 2014; Hosmer et al. 2011).

Inorganic nanoparticles have been extensively utilized due to their lower toxicity, better bioavailability compared with the free drug, and higher tolerance (Ketabat et al. 2019). Inorganic nanoparticles based on noble metals (e.g., silver, gold, and titanium) and iron oxide have been used in treatments, diagnostic and imaging processes. Their improved photo-thermal and highly controlled optical properties are important advantages and enable a high efficacy in therapeutic applications (El-Sayed, Huang, and El-Sayed 2006). These inorganic nanoparticles can target to a specific site by attaching the ligand to the nanoparticle, and higher photostability compared to organic dyes as well. However, the limited effective delivery due to limited penetration depth for photothermal therapy, and the inability to deliver biomacromolecules (e.g., proteins) are their main disadvantages (Ketabat et al. 2019).

Other systems based on inorganic nanoparticles have been proposed, such as mesoporous silica nanoparticles, and they displayed promising efficacy for anti-cancer therapy. Their biocompatibility, high porosity, and amenability for surface functionalization are suitable characteristics for the use in the treatment of OSCC (Ding et al. 2020; Wang et al. 2018; Shi et al. 2019). The porous characteristic of these particles enables to get much more free space for incorporation of antitumor drugs, and combined with polymers, they can carry active agents with high efficiency in targeting OSCC cells (Wang et al. 2018; Shi et al. 2019). However, additional studies are necessary for the routine implementation of these systems into clinical practice (Ketabat et al. 2019). The combinational nanoparticles have been also explored using polymeric and inorganic particles, such as using PLGA and silver nanoparticles. A study also confirmed that PLGA-silver nanoparticles containing the anticancer agent quinacrine inhibited proliferation of OSCC and reduced neo-angiogenesis, suggesting their promising application for the treatment of OSCC (Desai 2018; Satapathy et al. 2015).

Iron-oxide magnetic nanoparticles can be utilized together platforms for oral mucosal administration. After the local application of formulation, a magnetic field can be also applied and the magnetic energy can be transmitted to the nanoparticles in the form of heat, increasing the temperature of tumor tissue. Cancer cells can be selectively destroyed due to their more sensitivity to hyperthermia than healthy ones (Bruschi and Toledo 2019). For example, magnetite cationic liposomal particles and dextran-coated magnetite were utilized for the therapy of tumor cells by hyperthermia displaying promising results (Akbarzadeh et al. 2012). The selective magnetic hyperthermia can be restricted to the tumor area. In addition, the use of subdomain magnetic particles (nanometer-size particles) instead multidomain (micron-sized particles) enables the nanoparticles absorbing much more power at tolerable AC magnetic fields. Moreover, iron-oxide magnetic nanoparticles can deliver photosensitizers in PDT, using dextran coatings for prevention of nanoparticle aggregation and to allow for the linkage of hypericin. Therefore, it is possible to increase the selectivity and reduce the adverse effects of PDT (Unterweger et al. 2015).

Pharmaceutical dosage forms composed of cyclodextrin inclusion complexes are a group of systems with great potential for oral mucosal administration. Due to their chemical composition and structural special conformation (cyclical and composed of at least six units of glucose), cyclodextrins can enable bioavailability and multifunctional features, which can reduce the undesirable properties of active agents that are included in complexes. Therefore, the administration of these agents by oral mucosal route can be feasible.

Natural cyclodextrins (α-, β-, and γ-cyclodextrin) are utilized for the development of pharmaceutical systems and they show excellent biocompatibility, ability to improve the solubility and permeability, and mask undesirable organoleptic properties of drugs. Due to these cyclodextrins demonstrate limitations for the transport of active agents, enabling the loading of only lipophilic drugs, chemical modifications of them can be applied to make the cyclodextrins amphiphilic (Calixto et al. 2014). In this context, cyclodextrin complex can receive plasticizers, linoleic acid, zein, and hyaluronic acid for control the release of anticancer agents, such as paclitaxel (Esposito et al. 2020; Jing et al. 2013).

Many of these systems can be combined to result new final dosage forms with improved properties for oral mucosal administration, aiming the delivery of anticancer agents on OSCC treatment. For this, it is fundamental the understanding of physiochemical characteristics of drug, of system (and their composition and structure) and the oral mucosal environment.

Safety and Toxicity

These studies are quite important to confirm the efficacy of these formulations in terms of efficiency and security. The initial tests are performed *in vitro* and *in vivo*, and finally achieve the clinical trials (Ferreira et al. 2020).

In Vivo Evaluation

Most *in vivo* tests have been performed in polymeric nanoparticles, liposomes, hydrogel-based drug delivery systems, inorganic nanoparticles and nanorods, DNA- based nanostructures and nanoparticles and using other technologies containing anticancer agents testing in hamsters and mice (Calixto et al. 2014; Ketabat et al. 2019; Ding et al. 2020).

Cisplatin isolated and combined with a photosensitizer and naringenin have been incorporated in polymeric nanoparticles and their efficacy against OSCC have been investigated by different authors (Sulfikkarali et al. 2013; Endo et al. 2013; He, Liu, and Lin 2015). Polymeric nanoparticles containing cisplatin was studied by Endo and collaborators. They performed *in vivo* studies to evaluate the antitumor activity and found 4.4-6.6- fold higher antitumor activity in comparison to control group. When comparing the administration of cisplatin in solution, the polymeric nanoparticles were safer (decreased nephrotoxicity and neurotoxicity) (Endo et al. 2013). Coordination polymer – based core-shell nanoparticles containing cisplatin and pyrolipid (a photosensitizer) were evaluated by He and colleagues. They performed a cisplatin-resistant subcutaneous xenograft murine model and observed a notable tumor reduction of 83% after the treatment and irradiation (He, Liu, and Lin 2015). Sulfikkarali et al. (2013) evaluated the anti-tumor effects of naringenin-nanoparticles over 7,12-demethylbenz(a) anthracene-induced oral carcinogenesis and noticed an improved biochemical status (Sulfikkarali et al. 2013).

In vivo evaluation of liposomes has been investigated with the photodynamic therapy approach with the same formulation aluminum phthalocyanine chloride liposomes by the same authors in different works (Longo et al. 2009, 2012). They induced tongue carcinogenesis by ectopic transplantation of Ehrlich cancer cells (Longo et al. 2009) and topic 4-nitroquinoline-1-oxide (chemical carcinogenesis) in Swiss mice (Longo et al. 2012). Both studies showed the effectiveness of liposomes against oral cancer.

Two anticancer drugs (suberoylanilide hydroxamic acid and cisplatin) were loaded in a hydrogel for OSCC treatment, and the anticancer activity was evaluated in xenograft mice groups by Li and colleagues (2012). The treatment with the hydrogel loaded with the two drugs showed enhanced therapeutic effects and reduced side effects in comparison to the other groups (control, drugs isolated and cisplatin-loaded hydrogel (Li et al. 2012).

The *in vivo* assays were also performed in gold nanospheres and gold nanorods. Afifi and collaborators used gold nanospheres and the photothermal therapy approach (plasmonic method) for superficial OSCC treatment. Using OSCC hamster models, the gold nanospheres were injected followed by laser exposure. The outcomes revealed minimum adverse effects in healthy surrounding cells and sufficient short-term effects (Afifi et al. 2013). Wang et al. investigated the *in vivo* activity of gold nanorods loaded with rose Bengal in hamster models of oral cancer using photothermal therapy and photodynamic therapy isolated and combined (B.

Wang et al. 2014). The association of both therapeutic approaches enhanced singlet oxygen generation and increased uptake of photosensitizer.

Nucleoside-based drug delivery systems have been developed for OSCC treatment and the anticancer efficacy was studied in mouse xenograft model of OSCC. Zhao at al. developed self-assembled nucleoside nanoparticle loaded with 5-FU, which showed excellent anticancer efficacy in the *in vivo* models (Zhao et al. 2015).

Other technologies have been developed for human oral cancer treatment including near infrared excitable upconversion nanoparticles and microbubbles as carriers of siRNA (Lucky et al. 2016; Carson et al. 2012). Lucky and collaborators evaluated the anticancer activity of near-infrared excitable upconversion nanoparticle with photodynamic approach over xenograft tumor. Their outcomes revealed delay in tumor growth and improved survival rate and safety (Lucky et al. 2016). Carson et al. used a murine squamous cell carcinoma (SCC-VII) to assess the anticancer activity of microbubbles to the tumor site and found tumor growth suppression in mice (Carson et al. 2012).

In Vitro Evaluation

The *in vitro* evaluation of the cytotoxicity has been investigated in a wide range of nanostructured formulations including liposomes, inorganic nanoparticles and nanorods, combinational (polymeric- inorganic) nanoparticles, DNA-based nanoparticles, and semisolid systems (Calixto et al. 2014; Ketabat et al. 2019; Ding et al. 2020). Some of these studies have been performed in combination with diverse therapeutical approaches such as photodynamic therapy and photothermal therapy, which will be better explained in this session (Velloso et al. 2012; Longo et al. 2009; Bhana et al. 2016; Master et al. 2012; J. Li et al. 2012; B. Wang et al. 2014).

Liposomal carriers have been studies by diverse authors. Ayesa and collaborators (2017) performed the proliferation assay with lipid-soluble Zn (II)-bis-dipicolyllamine derivative cancer cells, which could eliminate the cells without anticancer drugs (Ayesa et al. 2017). Aluminum-phthalocyanine chloride liposomes were investigated to treated oral cancer cells with photodynamic therapy. Velloso and colleagues (2012) found that the aluminum-phthalocyanine chloride liposomes induced oral SCC death by inhibiting phosphatidylinositol 3-kinase/Akt/mammalian target of rapamycin signaling pathway (Velloso et al. 2012).

Polymeric nanoparticles containing traditional drugs (e.g., cisplatin), photosensitizers (e.g., chlorin - e6) and the active pharmaceutical ingredient curcumin (CUR) have been developed and used to treat OSCC cells. CUR-PLGA loaded nanoparticles have been studied by Chang and collaborators (2013) over the ability shock on Cal27- cisplatin resistant SCC cells. The authors found that nanoparticles containing CUR could induce cell apoptosis and inhibit cell growth in SCC cells by regulating the multiple drug resistance protein 1 (MDR1) and generating reactive oxygen species (Chang et al. 2013). In addition, polycaprolactone (PCL) nanoparticles coated with chitosan demonstrated the significant reduction of SCC-9 cell viability after the treatment (Mazzarino et al. 2015). Wang et al. 2015 prepared nanoparticles with PLGA and PEG with a wide range of drugs against OSCC and found efficient intracellular uptake of the nanoparticles (Wang et al. 2015). Master and colleagues (2012) showed that a hydrophobic photosensitizer Pc 4 incorporated in block-copolymer micelles could accelerate the cellular intracellular uptake in comparison to free photosensitizer (Master et al. 2012). The photosensitizer chlorin (e6)-loaded nanoparticles showed better *in vitro* photodynamic activity in comparison to free chlorin (e6) in Cal27 oral cancer cells (J. Li et al. 2012). Polymeric nanoparticles containing PEG-poly(glutamic acid) block copolymer and cisplatin were used to treat SCC-9 and induced apoptosis by activating caspase-3 and caspase-7 pathways (Endo et al. 2013). Sulfikkarali et at (2013) studied the anticancer effects of nanoparticles containing naringenin and found more intense effects in the naringenin loaded nanoparticles than free naringenin (Sulfikkarali et al. 2013).

Diverse inorganic nanoparticles and nanorods loaded with gold, iron and photosensitizers have been investigated for OSCC treatment. The investigation reported by Wu et al. (2011) found irreversible membrane-potential loss in mitochondria of OSCC cells after the treatment with iron core-gold shell nanoparticles. The authors suggested that these nanoparticles hindered the growth of oral cancer cells selectively by mitochondria-mediated autophagy (Wu et al. 2011). Nanospheres synthesized with N-rich mesoporous carbon were exposed to OSCC cells and internalized inducing thermal ablation effect on tumor (Das et al. 2019). Silicon 2,3-naphthalocyanine dihydroxide-loaded gold nanorods were investigated by Bhana et al. (2016) for photodynamic therapy and photothermal therapy simultaneously. The combined therapeutic approaches demonstrated improved activity in comparison to PDT or PTT alone (Bhana et al. 2016). This combined therapeutic approach was also reported by Wang et al. (2014), which studied rose Bengal loaded- gold nanorods and found improved outcomes over oral cancer cells with suitable singlet oxygen generation and better cellular uptake of photosensitizer (Wang et al. 2014). El-Sayed and collaborators (2005) developed anti-epithelial growth factor receptor (EGFR) antibody-conjugated gold (Au) nanoparticles and exposed them to OSCC cells to evaluate the photothermal destruction. Their outcomes revealed the improved photothermal destruction on OSCC cells over benign cells (El-Sayed, Huang, and El-Sayed 2006). Fe nanoparticles containing anticancer agents promoted the induction of cancer cell apoptosis with better outcomes that individual chemotherapy and magnetic guided delivery (Sato et al. 2016).

The use of combined polymeric and inorganic nanoparticles has been employed to decrease silver nanoparticles toxicity of healthy cells. Satapathy evaluated the efficiency of PLGA based quinacrine- silver hybrid nanoparticles and revealed higher cytotoxicity over cancer cells and reduced neo-angiogenesis. These outcomes suggest that this formulation could be promising for OSCC treatment (Satapathy et al. 2015).

DNA-based nanoparticles and nanostructures have been also studied for OSCC treatment using *in vitro* studies. The anticancer aptamer AS141 was used to investigate the drug-delivery ability and tumor targeting and showed improved drug delivery and anticancer effects with fewer impacts in normal cells (Q. Li et al. 2017). In addition, monomeric self-assembled nucleoside nanoparticles were developed and have been loaded with 5-fluoroacil. *In vitro* studies confirmed the biocompatibility and low toxicity of these formulations.

In vitro studies with semisolid formations (gel and emulgel) have also been explored to deliver curcumin. CUR-loaded polymer blends were evaluated over Cal-26, FaDu cells and healthy keratinocytes and showed selectivity for cancer cells (Ferreira et al. 2019). In addition, the efficacy of CUR-loaded emulgels was tested in monolayers and tissue-engineered models, confirming the selectivity of curcumin for these cancer cells (Ferreira et al. 2020).

Clinical Trials

The clinical trials display huge importance in the development of new drug delivery system for OSCC treatment to guarantee the safety and efficacy. However, it was found few clinical studies testing formulations for OSCC treatment.

Basak and co-authors (2020) investigated Phase I on APG-157 oral delivered pastille (combination of CUR related polyphenol molecules with 100 mg drug substance) to assess the potential use as an oral drug for OSCC treatment. This was a double-blind, randomized and placebo-controlled clinical trial, where 25 subjects were recruited (12 patients with oral cancer and 13 normal control volunteers). In the normal control groups, 4 individuals received 100-mg placebo group, 3 individuals taken 100-mg APG-157 drug, 2 taken 200 mg placebo group and 4 received 200-mg APG157 treatment while for the oral cancer volunteers, 2 received 100-mg placebo group, 3 received 100-mg APG-157 treatment, 4 taken 200-mg placebo group and 3 received 200-mg APG-157 treatment. The patients were taken the drug orally by two different doses (3x100 mg and 3x200 mg) each hour, during three consecutive hours. Blood and saliva were collected, and expression of cytokines was analyzed before the treatment and after 1, 2, 3, and 24 hours of treatment. In addition, tumor biopsies were taken prior and post-treatment to evaluate the expression of RNAseq and immunofluorescence. The inflammatory cytokines, IL-1β, TNF-α, IL-8 were inhibition in a dose-dependent way of cancer patients treated with the drug. In addition, gene ontologies of cell cycle, cell adhesion and cell division were downregulated after the treatment, as well as it was observed an increase of CD4, CD8 T cells suggesting that APG-157 may be used as an adjuvant treatment (Basak et al. 2020).

The perioral cancer submucosal injection of curcubatacin BE polylactic acid nanoparticles were tested for delivery to cervical lymph nodes. The outcomes revealed higher drug concentrations than control group and lower blood concentrations than control group (Yang et al., 2003).

Two clinical trials testing freeze-dried raspberry lozenges in preventing oral cancer recurrence at oral cancer survivors and paclitaxel albumin stabilized nanoparticle formulation followed by chemoradiation in treating patients with recurrent head and neck cancer are in progress. So, there are no available results (Chicago 2021; Center 2020).

Patents and Market

The mucosal linings of the oral cavity can offer distinct advantages over parenteral and per oral administration for anticancer drugs, as previously described. The demand for oral mucosa as potential release and drug absorption site is obvious.

Considering the various strategies discussed, as well as the technologies that can be applied, many pharmaceutical systems for oral mucosal administration on OSCC treatment have been investigated.

These systems can be designed in different dosage forms, since their properties are dependent of the futures of the materials utilized during their preparation. In this context, the search for new materials, technologies and innovation is a constant.

The patent registration of a pharmaceutical system for buccal mucosal administration for the treatment of OSCC should consider the novelty and usefulness of the purpose.

The platform and system's value as hierarchical is particularly important. During the patent term period, nobody can use the pharmaceutical formulation for any purpose without the holder's permission.

Many dosage forms displaying different chemical compositions and technologies were developed and patents were deposited. Patents were deposited comprising solid and semisolid mucoadhesive systems composed of synthetic polymers (e.g., Carbomers, polyvinylpyrrolidone, polyvinylalcohol, polycarbophil, polyacrylate and/or polymethacrylate, polyethylene oxide polymers, polyethers, sulfate-functionalized polymers, amine-functionalized polymers, poly(2-alkyl-2-oxazoline), maleic acid copolymers, Eudragit RS, platinum-based brush-arm star polymers), gelatin, dextran, arabinogalactan, pullulan, hyaluronic acid, pectins, starch derivatives, cyclodextrins, alginates, chitosan, cellulose derivatives, gums and other polysaccharides (Zerbe, 2011; Domb and Wolnerman 2011; Constantini and Lemarchand 2011; Nystrom and Bredenberg 2011; Jolly 2012; Whitehead et al. 2012; Harris et al. 2013; Aiache et al. 2013; Attali et al. 2013; Sainti-lu et al. 2014; Whittle and Guy 2011; Feldstein et al. 2011; Quaglia et al. 2013; Boudy et al. 2014; Mallery et al. 2014; Malcovati et al. 2011; Vasisht and Finn 2011; Evans et al. 2011; Loewy et al. 2012; Longo 2013; Schwab et al. 2014; Caramela et al. 2011; Botoni et al. 2013; Johnson and Liao 2018). Tablets, emulsion systems, gels, films or patches, and liquid colloidal dispersions are the main final dosage forms found.

In this context, there are there are thousands of applications and patents granted showing formulations. The market is promissory; however, there is a relatively much smaller number of medicines already available on the market.

It is clear the necessity for new and suitable medicines for buccal mucosal administration aiming the chemoprevention and therapy of OSCC. For this the improvement of the mechanistic understanding of OSCC is very important (Ketabat et al. 2019; Sarma et al. 2019).

CONCLUSION

The main objective of cancer treatment is the selective total killing of cancer cells, avoiding side effects. Therefore, improvements of drug targeting to specific places in the body to achieve defined therapeutic effects are necessary. When the aim is the buccal mucosal administration of pharmaceutical systems, the knowledge of the characteristics of this particular environment, materials and strategies to be utilized is fundamental. Therefore, efforts have been done for the development of suitable technologies and new materials.

The smooth and relatively immobile surface of the buccal mucosa enables the development pharmaceutical dosage form for sustained delivery of anti-cancer agents. Mucoadhesive dosage forms have many advantages over traditional oral ones, enabling a prolonged residence time and improving the drug bioavailability.

Drug delivery systems for oral mucosal administration in the OSCC treatment consist of the anticancer agents (single or multiple), carriers as platforms for the agents, and the strategies of drug delivery to the tumor cells. The platforms can be composed of materials from natural, synthetic, or semi-synthetic origin, and different solid and semi-solid systems have been proposed for the oral mucosal administration in OSCC treatment and the choice of better also depends on the characteristics of the bioactive agent. In this sense, those displaying short biological half-lives, require sustained delivery.

The use of nanotechnology is an important strategy for overcoming encountered obstacles to efficiently target several cancers cell types, leading to the optimal anti-oral tumor effects. Many advances were achieved; however, further investigations are needed to improve the practical applications.

The advent of personalized medicine may lead to the improved therapeutic outcomes of OSCC. In addition, lower cost treatments and the increase of survival rates can be reached as important gains for both patients and therapeutics in a next future.

The biological *in vivo* and *in vitro* tests are particularly important to evaluate the performance of these drug delivery systems. Animal models have been used as *in vivo* investigation, and they are performed with xenograft and chemically induced- tumors. *In vitro* studies have been carried out with cell culture (malignant and healthy cells) and tissue-engineered models. Despite the clinical trials are the most important to predict safety and efficacy of these drug delivery systems, there are few finalized studies.

References

Adelstein, David J., Li, Y., Adams, G. L., Wagner, H., Kish, J. A., Ensley, J. F., Schuller, D. E. and Forastiere, A. A. (2003). An Intergroup Phase III Comparison of Standard Radiation Therapy and Two Schedules of Concurrent Chemoradiotherapy in Patients with Unresectable Squamous Cell Head and Neck Cancer. *Journal of Clinical Oncology,* 21 (1), 92–98.

Afifi, M. M., El Sheikh, S. M., Abdelsalam, M. M., Ramadan, H., Omar, T. A., El Tantawi, M., Abdel-Razek, K. M., and Mohamed M. (2013). Therapeutic Efficacy of Plasmonic Photothermal Nanoparticles in Hamster Buccal Pouch Carcinoma. *Oral Surgery, Oral Medicine, Oral Pathology and Oral Radiology,* 115 (6), 743–751.

Agüeros, M., Ruiz-Gatón, L., Vauthier, C., Bouchemal, K., Espuelas, S., Ponchel, G., and Irache, J. M. (2009). Combined Hydroxypropyl-β-Cyclodextrin and Poly(Anhydride) Nanoparticles Improve the Oral Permeability of Paclitaxel. *European Journal of Pharmaceutical Sciences,* 38 (4), 405–413.

Aiache, J.-M., Constantini, D., Chaumont, C. (2013). *Prolonged release bioadhesive therapeutic systems.* US0310335A1.

Akbarzadeh, A., Samiei, M. and Davaran, S. (2012). Magnetic nanoparticles: Preparation, physical properties, and applications in biomedicine. *Nanoscale Res. Lett.*,7, 144.

Almeida, H., Amaral, M. H., Lobão, P., and Lobo J. M. S. (2013). In Situ Gelling Systems: A Strategy to Improve the Bioavailability of Ophthalmic Pharmaceutical Formulations. *Drug Discovery Today* 00 (00).

Alvarez-Lorenzo, C., Bromberg, L., Concheiro, A. (2009). Review lightsensitive intelligent drug delivery systems. *Source Doc Photobiol*, 85, 848-860.

Anaya, M. M., Franco, J. V. A., Ballesteros, M., Solà, I, Cuchí, G. U. and Cosp, X. B. (2019). Evidence Mapping and Quality Assessment of Systematic Reviews on Therapeutic Interventions for Oral Cancer. *Cancer Management and Research,* 11, 117–130.

Andrews, G. P., Laverty, T. P. and Jones, D. S. (2009). Mucoadhesive Polymeric Platforms for Controlled Drug Delivery. *European Journal of Pharmaceutics and Biopharmaceutics,* 71 (3), 505–518.

Attali, P., Lemarchand, C., Roulet, V., Scheuir, C., Zakin, L. (2013). *Treating inflammation and inflammatory pain in mucosa using mucosal prolonged release bioadhesive therapeutic carriers*. US0274306A1.

Ayesa, U., Gray, B. D., Pak, K. Y. and Chong, P. L. G. (2017). Liposomes Containing Lipid-Soluble Zn(II)-Bis-Dipicolylamine Derivatives Show Potential to Be Targeted to Phosphatidylserine on the Surface of Cancer Cells. *Molecular Pharmaceutics,* 14 (1), 147–156.

Basak, S. K., Bera, A., Yoon, A. J., Morselli, M., Jeong, C., Tosevska, A., Dong, T. S., et al. (2020). A Randomized, Phase 1, Placebo-Controlled Trial of APG-157 in Oral Cancer Demonstrates Systemic Absorption and an Inhibitory Effect on Cytokines and Tumor-Associated Microbes. *Cancer,* 126 (8), 1668–1682.

Bassi da Silva, J., de Souza Ferreira, S. B., de Freitas, O. and Bruschi, M. L. (2017). A Critical Review about Methodologies for the Analysis of Mucoadhesive Properties of Drug Delivery Systems. *Drug Development and Industrial Pharmacy,* 43 (7), 1053–1070.

Batrakova, E. V., and Kim, M. S. (2015). Using Exosomes, Naturally-Equipped Nanocarriers, for Drug Delivery. *Journal of Controlled Release,* 219, 396–405.

Bhana, S., O'Connor, R., Johnson, J., Ziebarth, J. D., Henderson, L. and Huang, X. (2016). Photosensitizer-Loaded Gold Nanorods for near Infrared Photodynamic and Photothermal Cancer Therapy. *Journal of Colloid and Interface Science,* 469, 8–16.

Bikram M. and West J. L. (2008). Thermo-responsive systems for controlled drug delivery. *Expert Opin Drug Deliv*, 5(10), 1077-1091.

Boiy, A., Roelandts, R. and de Witte, P. A. M. (2011). Photodynamic therapy using topically applied hypericin: comparative effect with methylaminolevulinic acid on UV induced skin tumours. *J Photochem Photobiol B*, 102(2), 123-131.

Bomeli, S. R., Desai, S. C., Johnson, J. T. and Walvekar, R. R. (2008). Management of Salivary Flow in Head and Neck Cancer Patients - A Systematic Review. *Oral Oncology,* 44 (11),1000–1008.

Bonner, J. A., Harari, P. M., Giralt, J., Cohen, R. B., Jones, C. U., Sur, R. K., Raben, D., et al. (2010). Radiotherapy plus Cetuximab for Locoregionally Advanced Head and Neck Cancer: 5-Year Survival Data from a Phase 3 Randomised Trial, and Relation between Cetuximab-Induced Rash and Survival. *The Lancet Oncology,* 11 (1), 21–28.

Bottoni, G., Maffei, P., Sforzini, A., Federici, M., Caramella, C., Rossi, S. and Viscomi, G. C. (2013). *Mucoadhesive xyloglucan-containing formulationsuseful inmedical devices and in pharmaceutical fromulations*. US0183325A1.

Boudy, V., Tibi, A., D'Hayer, B., Husson, M. C. and Graff de Faget, S. (2014). *Gellin formulation containing ketamine*. WO033680A1.

Brannon-Peppas, L. and Blanchette J. O. (2012). Nanoparticle and targeted systems for cancer therapy. *Adv Drug Deliv Rev.* 64, 206–212.

Brewer, E., Coleman, J. and Lowman A. (2011). Emerging technologies of polymeric nanoparticles in cancer drug delivery. *J Nanomater.* (2011), 408675.

Bruschi, M. L. (2015). Mathematical Models of Drug Release. In *Strategies to Modify the Drug Release from Pharmaceutical Systems*, M. L. Bruschi (Eds.), First, 1:63–86. Sawston: Woodhead Publishing.

Bruschi, M. L. and Toledo L. A. S. (2019) Pharmaceutical applications of iron-oxide magnetic nanoparticles. *Magnetochemistry*. 5(50), 1-19.

Bruschi, M. L., and de Freitas, O. (2005). Oral Bioadhesive Drug Delivery Systems. *Drug Development and Industrial Pharmacy* 31: 293–310.

Bruschi, M. L., Bassi da Silva, J. and Rosseto, H. C. (2019). Photodynamic therapy of psoriasis using photosensitizers of vegetable origin. *Curr Pharm Des*, 25,1-13.

Bruschi, M. L., Borghi-Pangoni, F. B., Junqueira, M. V., and de Souza Ferreira, S. B. (2017). Nanostructured Therapeutic Systems with Bioadhesive and Thermoresponsive Properties. D. Ficai and A. M. Grumezescu (Eds.). *Nanostructures for Novel Therapy: Synthesis, Characterization and Applications*. Amsterdam: Elsevier Inc.

Bruschi, M. L., Borghi-Pangoni, F. B., Junqueira, M. V., de Souza Ferreira, S. B. and da Silva, J. B. (2017). Environmentally Responsive Systems for Drug Delivery. *Recent Patents on Drug Delivery and Formulation,* 11, (2).

Bruschi, M. L., de Freitas, O., Lara, E. H. G., Panzeri, H., Gremião, M. P. D. and Jones, D. S. (2008). Precursor System of Liquid Crystalline Phase Containing Propolis Microparticles for the Treatment of Periodontal Disease: Development and Characterization. *Drug Development and Industrial Pharmacy,* 34 (3), 267–278.

Bruschi, M. L., De Souza Ferreira, S. B. and Bassi da Silva, J. (2020). Mucoadhesive and Mucus-Penetrating Polymers for Drug Delivery. In *Nanotechnology for Oral Drug Delivery: From Concept to Applications*, J. P. Martins and H. A. Santos (Eds.), First, 77–123. London: Academic Press.

Bunggulawa, E. J., Wang, W., Yin, T., Wang, N., Durkan, C., Wang, Y. and Wang, G. (2018). Recent Advancements in the Use of Exosomes as Drug Delivery Systems 06 Biological Sciences 0601 Biochemistry and Cell Biology. *Journal of Nanobiotechnology,* 16 (1), 1–13.

Burki, I. K., Khan, M. K., Khan, B. A., Uzair, B., Braga, V. A. and Jamil, Q. A. (2020). Formulation Development, Characterization, and Evaluation of a Novel Dexibuprofen-Capsaicin Skin Emulgel with Improved *In Vivo* Anti-inFl Ammatory and Analgesic Effects. *AAPS Pharm Sci Tech,* 21, 1–14.

Calixto, G., Bernegossi, J., Fonseca-Santos, B. and Chorilli, M. (2014)). Nanotechnology-Based Drug Delivery Systems for Treatment of Oral Cancer: A Review. *International Journal of Nanomedicine,* 9 (1), 3719–3735.

Capote-Moreno, A., Brabyn, P., Muñoz-Guerra, M. F., Sastre-Pérez, J., Escorial-Hernandez, V., Rodríguez-Campo, F. J., García, T. and Naval-Gías, L. (2020). Oral Squamous Cell Carcinoma: Epidemiological Study and Risk Factor Assessment Based on a 39-Year Series. *International Journal of Oral and Maxillofacial Surgery,* 49 (12), 1525–1534.

Caramella, C. M., Bonferoni, M. C., Rossi, S. S., Sandri, G., Ferrari, F., Perotti, C. G. and Fante, C. D. (2011). *Platelet lysate and bioadhesive compositions thereof for the treatment of mucositis*. US0280952A1.

Carson, A. R., McTiernan, C. F., Lavery, L., Grata, M., Leng, X., Wang, J., Chen, X. and Villanueva, F. S. (2012). Ultrasound-Targeted Microbubble Destruction to Deliver SiRNA Cancer Therapy. *Cancer Research,* 72 (23), 6191–6199.

Carvalho, F. C., Bruschi, M. L., Evangelista, R. C., Gremião, M. P. D., Shaikh, R., Singh, T. R. R., Garland, M. J., Woolfson, A. D. and Donnelly, R. F. (2010). Mucoadhesive Drug Delivery Systems. *Brazilian Journal of Pharmaceutical Sciences,* 46 (1), 1–18.

Center, Ohio State University Comprehensive Cancer. (2020). "Freeze-Dried Black Raspberries in Preventing Oral Cancer Recurrence in High At-Risk Appalachian Patients Oral Cancer Survivors." *Clinical Trials*. Acessed in: https://clinicaltrials.gov/ct2/show/study/NCT01504932 ?term=formulation&cond=Oral+Cancer&draw=2&
rank=1.

Chandran, P., Sasidharan, A., Ashokan, A., Menon, D., Nair, S. and Koyakutty, M. (2011). Highly Biocompatible TiO_2:$Gd3^+$ Nano-Contrast Agent with Enhanced Longitudinal Relaxivity for Targeted Cancer Imaging. *Nanoscale,* 3 (10), 4150–4161.

Chang, P. Y., Peng, S. F., Lee, C. Y., Lu, C. C., Tsai, S. C., Shieh, T. M., Wu, T. S., Tu, M. G., Chen, M. Y. and Yang, J. S. (2013). Curcumin-Loaded Nanoparticles Induce Apoptotic Cell Death through Regulation of the Function of MDR1 and Reactive Oxygen Species in Cisplatin-Resistant CAR Human Oral Cancer Cells. *International Journal of Oncology,* 43 (4), 1141–1150.

Chiappin, S., Antonelli, G., Gatti, R. and De Palo, E. F. (2007). Saliva Specimen: A New Laboratory Tool for Diagnostic and Basic Investigation. *Clinica Chimica Acta,* 383 (1–2), 30–40.

Chicago, University of. (2021). Paclitaxel Albumin-Stabilized Nanoparticle Formulation and Carboplatin Followed By Chemoradiation in Treating Patients With Recurrent Head and Neck Cancer. *Clinical Trials.*

Acessed in: https://clinicaltrials.gov/ct2/show/record/NCT01847326 ?term=formulation&cond=Oral+Cancer&draw=2&rank=6.

Chidambaram, N., and Srivatsava, A. K. (1995). Buccal Drug Delivery Systems. *Drug Dev. Ind. Pharm,* 21 (9), 1009–1036.

Choudhary, S., Nouri, K. and Elsaie M. L. (2009. Photodynamic therapy in dermatology: a review. *Lasers Med Sci*. 24(6), 971-980.

Chu, K. S., Schorzman, A. N. and Finniss MC, et al. (2013). Nanoparticle drug loading as a design parameter to improve docetaxel pharmacokinetics and efficacy. *Biomaterials*. 34(33), 8424–8429.

Colley, H. E., Hearnden, V., Avila-Olias, M., Cecchin, D., Canton, I., Madsen, J., Macneil, S., et al. (2014). Polymersome-Mediated Delivery of Combination Anticancer Therapy to Head and Neck Cancer Cells: 2D and 3D *in Vitro* Evaluation. *Molecular Pharmaceutics,* 11 (4), 1176–1188.

Cook, M. T. and Vitaliy V. Khutoryanskiy. (2015). Mucoadhesion and Mucosa-Mimetic Materials—A Mini-Review. *International Journal of Pharmaceutics,* 495 (2), 991–998.

Costantini, D. and Lemarchand, C. (2011) *Compressed granulated mucosal bioadhesive slow release carrier for delivering active principles.* NZ571156A.

Das, R. K., Panda, S., Bhol, C. S., Bhutia, S. K. and Mohapatra, S. (2019). N-Doped Carbon Quantum Dot (NCQD)-Deposited Carbon Capsules for Synergistic Fluorescence Imaging and Photothermal Therapy of Oral Cancer. *Langmuir,* 35 (47), 15320–15329.

Desai, K. G. H. (2018). Polymeric Drug Delivery Systems for Intraoral Site-Specific Chemoprevention of Oral Cancer. *Journal of Biomedical Materials Research - Part B Applied Biomaterials,* 106 (3), 1383–1413.

Devalapally, H., Chakilam, A. and Amiji, M. M. (2006). Role of Nanotechnology in Pharmaceutical Product Development. *Journal of Pharmaceutical Sciences,* 96 (10), 2547–2565.

Dhanda, D. S., Tyagi, P., Mirvish, S. S. and Kompella, U. B. (2013). Supercritical fluid technology based large porous celecoxib-PLGA microparticles do not induce pulmonary fibrosis and sustain drug delivery and efficacy for several weeks following a single dose. *J Control Release*. 168(3), 239–250.

Ding, Z., Sigdel, K., Yang, L., Liu,Y., Xuan, M., Wang, X., Gu, Z., Wu, J. and Xie, H. (2020). Nanotechnology-Based Drug Delivery Systems for Enhanced Diagnosis and Therapy of Oral Cancer. *Journal of Materials Chemistry B,* 8 (38), 8781–8793.

Dissanayaka, W. L., Pitiyage, G., Kumarasiri, P. V. R., Liyanage, P. L. M. R., Dias, K. D. and Tilakaratne, W. M. (2012). Clinical and Histopathologic Parameters in Survival of Oral Squamous Cell Carcinoma. *Oral Surgery, Oral Medicine, Oral Pathology and Oral Radiology,* 113 (4), 518–525.

Domb, A. J. and Wolnerman, J. S. (2011). *Absorbable solid composition for topical treatment of oral mucosal disorders*. US0244039A1.

El-Sayed, I. H., Huang, X. and El-Sayed, M. A. (2006). Selective Laser Photo-Thermal Therapy of Epithelial Carcinoma Using Anti-EGFR Antibody Conjugated Gold Nanoparticles. *Cancer Letters,* 239 (1), 129–135.

Endo, K., Ueno, T., Kondo, S., Wakisaka, N., Murono, S., Ito, M., Kataoka, K., Kato, Y. and Yoshizaki, T. (2013). Tumor-Targeted Chemotherapy with the Nanopolymer-Based Drug NC-6004 for Oral Squamous Cell Carcinoma. *Cancer Science,* 104 (3), 369–374.

Esposito, D., Conte, C., d'Angelo, I., Miro, A., Ungaro, F. and Quaglia, F. (2020). Mucoadhesive Zein/Beta-Cyclodextrin Nanoparticles for the Buccal Delivery of Curcumin. *International Journal of Pharmaceutics,* 586 (May), 119587.

Evans, A. M., Song, Y. and Rao, S. (2011). *Novel drug delivery system.* WO137491A1.

Fan, W., Yan, W., Xu, Z. and Ni H. (2012). Formation mechanism of monodisperse, low molecular weight chitosan nanoparticles by ionic gelation technique. *Colloids Surf B Biointerfaces*. 90, 21–27.

Fang, J. Y., Fang, C. L., Liu, C. H. and Su Y. H. (2008). Lipid nanoparticles as vehicles for topical psoralen delivery: solid lipid nanoparticles (SLN) versus nanostructured lipid carriers (NLC). *Eur J Pharm Biopharm.* 70(2), 633–640.

Feldstein, M. M., Cleary, G., Kulichikhin, V. G., Bairamov, D. F. (2011). *Two-phase, water-absorbent bioadhesive compostion*. EP2277556A1.

Ferreira, S. B. S., Braga, G., Oliveira, E. L., da Silva, J. B., Rosseto, H. C., Hoshino, L. V. C., Baesso, M. L., et al. (2019). Design of a Nanostructured Mucoadhesive System Containing Curcumin for Buccal Application: From Physicochemical to Biological Aspects. *Beilstein Journal of Nanotechnology* 10, 2304–2328.

Ferreira, S. B. S., Slowik, K. M., Hoshino, L. V. C., Baesso, M. L., Murdoch, C., Colley, H. E. and Bruschi, M. L. (2020). Mucoadhesive Emulgel Systems Containing Curcumin for Oral Squamous Cell Carcinoma Treatment: From Pre-Formulation to Cytotoxicity in Tissue-Engineering Oral Mucosa. *European Journal of Pharmaceutical Sciences,* 151 (March), 105372.

Fong, W. -K., Negrini, R., Vallooran, J. J., Mezzenga, R. and Boyd B. J. (2016). Responsive self-assembled nanostructured lipid systems for drug delivery and diagnostics. *J Colloid Interface Sci*. 484, 320-339.

Fonseca-Santos, B. and Chorilli, M. (2018). An Overview of Polymeric Dosage Forms in Buccal Drug Delivery: State of Art, Design of Formulations and Their *in Vivo* Performance Evaluation. *Materials Science and Engineering C,* 86, 129–143.

Freitas, C., Müller, R. H. (1998). Effect of light and temperature on zeta potential andphysical stability in solid lipid nanoparticle (SLNTM) dispersions, *Int. J. Pharm*, 168, 221–229.

Gatta, G., Botta, L., Sánchez, M. J., Anderson, L. A., Pierannunzio, D., Licitra, L., Hackl, M., et al. (2015). Prognoses and Improvement for Head and Neck Cancers Diagnosed in Europe in Early 2000s: The EUROCARE-5 Population-Based Study. *European Journal of Cancer,* 51 (15), 2130–2143.

Ghanizada, M., Jakobsen, K. M., Grønhøj, C. and von Buchwald C. (2019). The Effects of Checkpoint Inhibition on Head and Neck Squamous Cell Carcinoma: A Systematic Review. *Oral Oncology,* 90 (January), 67–73.

Gowthamarajan, K., Jawahar, N., Wake, P., Jain, K. and Sood, S. (2012). Development of Buccal Tablets for Curcumin Using Anacardium Occidentale Gum. *Carbohydrate Polymers,* 88 (4), 1177–1183.

Guo, R., Peng, H., Tian, Y., Shen, S. and Yang, W. (2016). Mitochondria-Targeting Magnetic Composite Nanoparticles for Enhanced Phototherapy of Cancer. *Small (Weinheim an Der Bergstrasse, Germany),* 12 (33), 4541–4552.

Guo, Y.-g. and Singh, A. P. (2019). Emerging Strategies for Enhancing Buccal and Sublingual Administration of Nutraceuticals and Pharamaceuticals. *Journal of Drug Delivery Science and Technology,* 52, 440–451.

Ha, D., Yang, N. and Nadithe, V. (2016). Exosomes as therapeutic drug carriers and delivery vehicles across biological membranes: current perspectives and future challenges. *Acta Pharm. Sin. B.* 6, 287–296.

Hafizi, M., Kalanaky, S., Moaiery, H., Khayamzadeh, M., Noorian, S., Kaveh, V., Gharib, B., et al. (2019). A Randomized, Double-Blind, Placebo-Controlled Investigation of BCc1 Nanomedicine Effect on Survival and Quality of Life in Metastatic and Non-Metastatic Gastric Cancer Patients." *Journal of Nanobiotechnology,* 17 (1), 1–19.

Harris., B. Z., Murthy, V. M. K., Steinberg, D. A., Pearlmen, R., Rosen, H. B., Langer, R. S. and Barash, H. E. (2013). *Mucoadhesive devices for delivery of active agents*. WO188819A2.

He, C., Liu, D. and Lin, W. (2015). Self-Assembled Core-Shell Nanoparticles for Combined Chemotherapy and Photodynamic Therapy of Resistant Head and Neck Cancers. *ACS Nano,* 9 (1), 991–1003.

Holpuch, A. S., Hummel, G. J., Tong, M., et al. (2010). Nanoparticles for local drug delivery to the oral mucosa: proof of principle studies. *Pharm Res*. 27(7), 1224–1236.

Hosmer, J. M., Shin, S. H., Nornoo, H., Zheng, H. and Lopes, L. (2011). Influence of Internal Structure and Composition of Liquid Crystalline Phases on Topical Delivery of Paclitaxel. *Journal of Pharmaceutical Sciences,* 100 (4), 1444–1455.

Hsu, H. W., Wall, N. R., Hsueh, C. T., Kim, S., Ferris, R. L., Chen, C. S. and Mirshahidi S. (2014). Combination Antiangiogenic Therapy and Radiation in Head and Neck Cancers. *Oral Oncology,* 50 (1), 19–26.

Jiang, X. C. and Gao, J. Q. (2017). Exosomes as Novel Bio-Carriers for Gene and Drug Delivery. *International Journal of Pharmaceutics,* 521 (1–2), 167–175.

Jing, J., Szarpak-Jankowska, A., Guillot, R., Pignot-Paintrand, I., Picart, C. and Auzély-Velty, R. (2013). Cyclodextrin/Paclitaxel Complex in Biodegradable Capsules for Breast Cancer Treatment. *Chemistry of Materials,* 25 (19), 3867–3873.

Johnson, J. A. and Liao L. (2018). *Drug delivery polymer and uses thereof.* US10799594B2.

Jolly, J. F. (2012). *Controlled release formulations of enzymes, microorganisms, and antibodies with mucoadhesive polymers.* EP2422804A1.

Kaae, J. K., Stenfeldt, L. and Eriksen, J. G. (2016). Xerostomia after Radiotherapy for Oral and Oropharyngeal Cancer: Increasing Salivary Flow with Tasteless Sugar-Free Chewing Gum. *Frontiers in Oncology*, 6 (MAY), 1–6.

Ketabat, F., Pundir, M., Mohabatpour, F., Lobanova, L., Koutsopoulos, S., Hadjiiski, L., Chen, X., Papagerakis, P. and Papagerakis, S. (2019). Controlled Drug Delivery Systems for Oral Cancer Treatment—Current Status and Future Perspectives. *Pharmaceutics,* 11 (7), 1–29.

Khullar, R., Kumar, D., Seth, N. and Saini, S. (2012). Formulation and Evaluation of Mefenamic Acid Emulgel for Topical Delivery. *Saudi Pharmaceutical Journal,* 20 (1), 63–67.

Khutoryanskiy, V. V. (2011). Advances in Mucoadhesion and Mucoadhesive Polymers. *Macromolecular Bioscience* 11 (6): 748–64.

Kovacevic, A., Savic, S., Vuleta, G., Müller, R. and Keck, C. (2011). Polyhydroxy surfactants for the formulation of lipid nanoparticles (SLN and NLC): effects on size, physical stability and particle matrix structure. *Int J Pharm*. 406(1–2), 163–172.

Krasodomska, O., Paolicelli, P., Cesa, S., Casadei, M. A. and Jungnickel, C. (2016). Protectionand viability of fruit seeds oils by nanostructured lipid carrier (NLC)nanosuspensions, *J. Colloid Interface Sci*, 479, 25–33.

Lalla, R. V., Treister, N., Sollecito, T., Schmidt, B., Patton, L. L., Mohammadi, K., Hodges, J. S. and Brennan, M. T. (2017). Oral

Complications at 6 Months after Radiation Therapy for Head and Neck Cancer. *Oral Diseases,* 23 (8), 1134–1143.

Li, J., Gong, C., Feng, X., Zhou, X., Xu, X., Xie, L., Wang, R., et al. (2012). Biodegradable Thermosensitive Hydrogel for SAHA and DDP Delivery: Therapeutic Effects on Oral Squamous Cell Carcinoma Xenografts. *PLoS ONE,* 7 (4), 2–9.

Li, Q., Zhao, D., Shao, X., Lin, S., Xie, X., Liu, M., Ma, W., Shi, S. and Lin, Y. (2017). Aptamer-Modified Tetrahedral DNA Nanostructure for Tumor-Targeted Drug Delivery. *ACS Applied Materials and Interfaces,* 9 (42), 36695–36701.

Loewy, Z. G., Levine, W. Z., Saffer, A. J. (2012) *Anti-inflammatory dissolvable film.* US0003292A1.

Longo, J. P. F., Lozzi, S. P. and Azevedo, R. B. (2011). Buccal cancer and Photodyanamic therapy as a therapeutical modality. *RGO - Revista Gaúcha de Odontologia,* 59, 51–57.

Longo, J. P. F., Lozzi, S. P., Simioni, A. R., Morais, P. C., Tedesco, A. C. and Azevedo, R. B. (2009). Photodynamic Therapy with Aluminum-Chloro-Phtalocyanine Induces Necrosis and Vascular Damage in Mice Tongue Tumors. *Journal of Photochemistry and Photobiology B: Biology,* 94 (2), 143–146.

Longo, J. P. F., Muehlmann, L. A., Velloso, N. V., Simioni, A. R., Lozzi, S. P., Cavalcanti, C. E. O., Tedesco, A. C. and Azevedo, R. B. (2012). Effects of Photodynamic Therapy Mediated by Liposomal Aluminumphthalocyanine Chloride on Chemically Induced Tongue Tumors. *Chemotherapy: Open Access,* 01 (02), 2–5.

Longo, S. (2013). *Edible slow dissolving film for treating oral ulcerations.* WO110809A1.

Luan, X., Sansanaphongpricha, K., Myers, I., Chen, H., Yuan, H. and Sun, D. (2017). Engineering exosomes as refined biological nanoplatforms for drug delivery. *Acta Pharmacol. Sin.* 38, 754–763.

Lucky, S. S., Idris, N. M., Huang, K., Kim, J., Li, Z., Thong, Z. S. P., Xu, R., Soo, K. C. and Zhang, Y. (2016). *In Vivo* Biocompatibility, Biodistribution and Therapeutic Efficiency of Titania Coated

Upconversion Nanoparticles for Photodynamic Therapy of Solid Oral Cancers. *Theranostics,* 6 (11), 1844–65.

Makadia, H. K. and Siegel, S. J. (2011). Poly lactic-co-glycolic acid (PLGA) as biodegradable controlled drug delivery carrier. *Polymers (Basel).* 3(3), 1377–1397.

Malcovati, L. (2011). *Cancer sore patch.* US0160634A1.

Mallery, S. R., Larsen, P. E., Stoner, G. D., Schwendeman, P. and Desai, K. G. (2014). *Controlled release mucoadhesive systems.* US0056949A1.

Mansuri, S., Kesharwani, P., Jain, K., Tekade, R. K. and Jain, N. K. K. (2016). Mucoadhesion: A Promising Approach in Drug Delivery System. *Reactive and Functional Polymers,* 100, 151–172.

Masood, F. (2016). Polymeric Nanoparticles for Targeted Drug Delivery System for Cancer Therapy. *Materials Science and Engineering C,* 60, 569–578.

Master, A. M., Qi, Y., Oleinick, N. L. and Gupta, A. S. (2012). EGFR-Mediated Intracellular Delivery of Pc 4 Nanoformulation for Targeted Photodynamic Therapy of Cancer: *In Vitro* Studies. *Nanomedicine: Nanotechnology, Biology, and Medicine,* 8 (5), 655–664.

Mathias, N. R. and Li L. (2012). Composition for enhancing absorption of a drug and method. US20120053130A1.

Mathiowitz E., Chickering III, D. E. and Lehr C.-L. (1999). *Bioadhesive drug delivery systems – Fundamentals, novel approaches, and development.* 670p.

Mazzarino, L., Loch-Neckel, G., Bubniak, L. S., Mazzucco, S., Santos-Silva, M. C., Borsali, R. and Lemos-Senna, E. (2015). Curcumin-Loaded Chitosan-Coated Nanoparticles as a New Approach for the Local Treatment of Oral Cavity Cancer. *Journal of Nanoscience and Nanotechnology* 15 (1): 781–791.

Meher, J. G., Tarai, M., Yadav, N. P., Patnaik, A., Mishra, P. and Yadav, K. S. (2013). Development and Characterization of Cellulose-Polymethacrylate Mucoadhesive Film for Buccal Delivery of Carvedilol. *Carbohydrate Polymers,* 96 (1), 172–180.

Mohanraj, V. J. and Chen Y. (2006). Nanoparticles – a review. *Tropical Journal of Pharmaceutical Research.* 5(1), 561–573.

Morales, J. O. and McConville, J. T. (2014). Novel Strategies for the Buccal Delivery of Macromolecules. *Drug Development and Industrial Pharmacy,* 40 (5), 579–590.

Morantes, S. J., Buitrago, D. M., Ibla, J. F., Garcia, Y. M., Lafaurie, G. I. and Parraga, J. E. (2017). Composites of Hydrogels and Nanoparticles: A Potential Solution to Current Challenges in Buccal Drug Delivery. In *Biopolymer-Based Composites*, S. Jana, S. Mait and S. Jana (Eds), 1st ed., 107–138. Woodhead Publishing.

Mortazavi, S. A. and Smart, J. D. (1993). An Investigation into the Role of Water Movement and Mucus Gel Dehydration in Mucoadhesion. *Journal of Controlled Release,* 25, 197–203.

Nagai, T. and Machida, Y. (1993). Buccal Delivery Systems Using Hydrogels. *Advanced Drug Delivery Reviews,* 11 (1–2), 179–191.

Narihira, K., Watanabe, A., Sheng, H., Endo, H., Feril, L. B., Irie, Y., Ogawa, K., et al. (2018). Enhanced Cell Killing and Apoptosis of Oral Squamous Cell Carcinoma Cells with Ultrasound in Combination with Cetuximab Coated Albumin Microbubbles. *Journal of Drug Targeting,* 26 (3), 278–288.

Nho, Y. C., Park, J. S. and Lim, Y. M. (2014). Preparation of Poly(Acrylic Acid) Hydrogel by Radiation Crosslinking and Its Application for Mucoadhesives. *Polymers,* 6, 890–898.

Nystrom, C. and Bredenberg, S. (2011). *Rapid-Acting pharmaceutical composition.* US0256229A1.

O'neill, V. J. and Twelves, C. J. (2002). Oral Cancer Treatment: Developments in Chemotherapy and Beyond. *British Journal of Cancer,* 87 (9), 933–937.

Palem, C. R., Battu, S. K., Maddineni, S., Gannu, R., Repka, M. A. and Yamsani, M. A. (2013). Oral Transmucosal Delivery of Domperidone from Immediate Release Films Produced via Hot-Melt Extrusion Technology. *Pharmaceutical Development and Technology,* 18 (1), 186–195.

Paranjpe, M., J. H. Finke, C. Richter, T. Gothsch, A. Kwade, S. Büttgenbach, C. C. Müller-Goymann, Physicochemical characterization of sildenafil-loadedsolid lipid nanoparticle dispersions (SLN) for pulmonary application, *Int. J. Pharm.* 476 (2014) 41–49.

Patel, V. F., Liu, F. and Brown, M. B. (2012). Modeling the Oral Cavity: *In Vitro* and *in Vivo* Evaluations of Buccal Drug Delivery Systems. *Journal of Controlled Release,* 161 (3), 746–756.

Peppas, N. A., Slaughter, B. V. and Kanzelberger, M. A. (2012). Hydrogels (p. 385-395). In: Matyjaszewski K, Möller M (Ed.). *Polymer Science: A comprehensive reference*. Elsevier: Amsterdam. 20, v. 9.

Pereira, L. J., Caputo, J. B., Castelo, P. M., Andrade, E. F., Marques, L. S., de Paiva, S. M., Pereira, S. M. and Pereira, C. V. (2015). Fisiología Oral y Calidad de Vida En Pacientes Con Cáncer. *Nutricion Hospitalaria*, 31 (5), 2161–2166. [Oral Physiology and Quality of Life in Cancer Patients. *Hospital Nutrition*]

Pérez-Herrero, E. and Fernández-Medarde, A. (2015). Advanced Targeted Therapies in Cancer: Drug Nanocarriers, the Future of Chemotherapy. *European Journal of Pharmaceutics and Biopharmaceutics,* 93 (March), 52–79.

Petros, R. A. and DeSimone, J. M. (2010). Strategies in the design of nanoparticles for therapeutic applications. *Nat Rev Drug Discov*. 9(8), 615–627.

Pinto, L. S. S., De Aguiar, F. C. A., Kowalski, L. P., Graner E. and Lopes, M. A. (2010). FAS and ErbB2 Expression in Early Local Recurrent Oral Cancer. *Journal of Oral Pathology and Medicine,* 39 (2), 176–181.

Puratchikody, A., Prasanth, V. V., Mathew, S. T. and Kumar, A. B. (2011). Buccal Drug Delivery: Past, Present and Future - A Review. *International Journal of Drug Delivery,* 1 (2), 171–184.

Quaglia, F., Marenzi, C., Rotonda, M. I., Sammartino, G., Miro, A. and Ungaro, F. (2013). *Bioadhesive polymer-based controlled-release systems, production process and clinical uses thereof.* US0287819A1.

Rathbone, M. J. (1996). Oral mucosal drug delivery. 440p.

Rosseto, H. C., Toledo, L. A. S., Francisco, L. M. B., Esposito, E., Lim, Y., Valacchi, G., Cortesi, R. and Bruschi, M. L. (2017). Nanostructured Lipid Systems Modified with Waste Material of Propolis for Wound

Healing: Design, in Vitro and *in Vivo* Evaluation. *Colloids and Surfaces B: Biointerfaces,* 158, 441–452.

Ruel-Gariépy, E. and Leroux, J.-C. (2004). In Situ-Forming Hydrogels—Review of Temperature-Sensitive Systems. *European Journal of Pharmaceutics and Biopharmaceutics,* 58 (2), 409–426.

Russo, E., Selmin, F., Baldassari, S., Gennari, C. G. M., Caviglioli, G., Cilurzo, F., Minghetti, P. and Parodi, B. (2016). A Focus on Mucoadhesive Polymers and Their Application in Buccal Dosage Forms. *Journal of Drug Delivery Science and Technology* 32, 113–125.

Sager, H. (2012). Solid dispersing vaccine composition for oral delivery. US0034305A1.

Sagiri, S. S., Singh, V. K., Kulanthaivel, S., Banerjee, I., Basak, I., Battachrya, M. K. and Pal, K. (2015). Stearate Organogel-Gelatin Hydrogel Based Bigels: Physicochemical, Thermal, Mechanical Characterizations and *in Vitro* Drug Delivery Applications. *Journal of the Mechanical Behavior of Biomedical Materials,* 43, 1–17.

Said, Zulfahmi. (2018). *Analysis of Corticosteroid Drug Delivery Using Using Tissue-Engineered Oral Mucosa for The the Treatment of Inflammatory Mucosal Diseases Zulfahmi Said.* University of Sheffield.

Sainti-Lu, N., Razafindratsita, A., Tourdot, S., Moingeon, P. and Van Overtvelt, L. (2014). *Mucoadhesive particulate formulation for inducing antigen-specific immune tolerance*. US0079795A1.

Salamat-Miller, N., Chittchang, M. and Johnston, T. M. (2005). The Use of Mucoadhesive Polymers in Buccal Drug Delivery. *Advanced Drug Delivery Reviews,* 57 (11), 1666–1691.

Samra, B., Tam, E., Baseri, B. and Shapira, I. (2018). Checkpoint Inhibitors in Head and Neck Cancer: Current Knowledge and Perspectives. *Journal of Investigative Medicine,* 66 (7), 1023–1030.

Sandri, G., Ruggeri, M., Rossi, S., Bonferoni, M. C., Vigani, B. and Ferrari, F. (2020). (Trans)Buccal Drug Delivery (pp. 242-267). In *Nanotechnology for Oral Drug Delivery: From Concept to Applications*. J. P. Martins and H. A. Santos (Eds.). London.

Sangeetha, S., Venkatesh, D. N., Krishan, P. N. and Saraswathi, R. (2010). Mucosa as a Route for Systemic Drug Delivery. *Research Journal of Pharmaceutical, Biological and Chemical Sciences* 1 (3), 178–187.

Sarma, H., Jahan, T. and Sharma, H. K. (2019). Progress in Drug and Formulation Development for the Chemoprevention of Oral Squamous Cell Carcinoma: A Review. *Rec Pat Drug Deliv Formul.* 13, 16-36.

Satapathy, S. R., Siddharth, S., Das, D., Nayak, A. and Kundu, C. N. (2015). Enhancement of Cytotoxicity and Inhibition of Angiogenesis in Oral Cancer Stem Cells by a Hybrid Nanoparticle of Bioactive Quinacrine and Silver: Implication of Base Excision Repair Cascade. *Molecular Pharmaceutics,* 12 (11), 4011–4025.

Satheesh Madhav, N. V., Semwal, R., Semwal, D. K. and Semwal, R. B. (2012). Recent Trends in Oral Transmucosal Drug Delivery Systems: An Emphasis on the Soft Palatal Route. *Expert Opinion on Drug Delivery,* 9 (6), 629–647.

Sato, I., Umemura, M., Mitsudo, K., Fukumura, H., Kim, J. H., Hoshino, Y., Nakashima, H., et al. (2016). Simultaneous Hyperthermia-Chemotherapy with Controlled Drug Delivery Using Single-Drug Nanoparticles. *Scientific Reports,* 6 (March), 1–12.

Schmaljohann, D. (2006). Thermo- and pH-responsive polymers in drug delivery. *Adv Drug Deliv Rev,* 58(15), 1655-1670.

Schwab, J. J., Raven, J. S., Liu, F. (2014). *Mucosal tissue adhesion via textured surface.* WO022657A1.

Scully C, editor. (2013) Cancer. In: *Oral and Maxillofacial Medicine: The Basis of Diagnosis and Treatment.* 3rd ed. New York: Churchill Livingstone Elsevier (pp. 204–217).

Shi, X. L., Li, Y., Zhao, L. M., Su, L. W. and Ding, G. (2019). Delivery of MTH1 inhibitor (TH287) and MDR1 siRNA via hyaluronic acid-based mesoporous silica nanoparticles for oral cancers treatment. *Colloids Surf. B Biointerfaces.* 173, 599–606.

Siegel R. A. (2014). Stimuli sensitive polymers and self-regulated drug delivery systems: A very partial review. *J Control Release*, 190, 337-351.

Silva, J. B. da, Ferreira, S. B. S., Reis, A. V., Cook, M. T. and Bruschi, M. L. (2018). Assessing Mucoadhesion in Polymer Gels: The Effect of Method Type and Instrument Variables. *Polymers,* 10 (3), 1–19.

Sledge, G. W. and Miller, K. D. (2003). Exploiting the Hallmarks of Cancer: The Future Conquest of Breast Cancer. *European Journal of Cancer,* 39 (12), 1668–1675.

Smart, J. D. (1993). Drug Delivery Using Buccal-Adhesive Systems. *Advanced Drug Delivery Reviews,* 11, 253–270.

Souza Ferreira, S. B. and Bruschi, M. L. (2021). Investigation of the Physicochemical Stability of Emulgels Composed of Poloxamer 407 and Different Oil Phases Using the Quality by Design Approach. *Journal of Molecular Liquids,* 332, 115856.

Souza Ferreira, S. B. de and Bruschi, M. L. (2019). Improving the Bioavailability of Curcumin: Is Micro/Nanoencapsulation the Key? *Therapeutic Delivery*, 10 (2).

Souza Ferreira, S. B. De, Moço, T. D., Borghi-Pangoni, F. B., Junqueira, M. V. and Bruschi, M. L. (2015). Rheological, Mucoadhesive and Textural Properties of Thermoresponsive Polymer Blends for Biomedical Applications. *Journal of the Mechanical Behavior of Biomedical Materials,* 55, 164–178.

Souza Ferreira, S. B., Braga, G., Oliveira, E. L., Rosseto, H. C., Hioka, N., Caetano, W., and Bruschi, M. L. (2020). Colloidal Systems Composed of Poloxamer 407, Different Acrylic Acid Derivatives and Curcuminoids: Optimization of Preparation Method, Type of Bioadhesive Polymer and Storage Conditions. *Journal of Drug Delivery Science and Technology,* 57 (February), 101686.

Srivastava, S., Mohammad, S., Pant, A. B., Mishra, P. R., Pandey, G., Gupta, S. and Farooqui, S. (2018). Co-Delivery of 5-Fluorouracil and Curcumin Nanohybrid Formulations for Improved Chemotherapy Against Oral Squamous Cell Carcinoma. *Journal of Maxillofacial and Oral Surgery* 17 (4): 597–610.

Sudhakar, Y., Kuotsu, K. and Bandyopadhyay, A. K. (2006). Buccal Bioadhesive Drug Delivery - A Promising Option for Orally Less Efficient Drugs. *Journal of Controlled Release,* 114 (1), 15–40.

Sulfikkarali, N., Krishnakumar, N., Manoharan, S. and Nirmal, R. M. (2013). Chemopreventive Efficacy of Naringenin-Loaded Nanoparticles in 7,12-Dimethylbenz(a)Anthracene Induced Experimental Oral Carcinogenesis. *Pathology and Oncology Research,* 19 (2), 287–296.

Sun, D., Zhuang, X., Xiang, X., Liu, Y., Zhang, S., Liu, C., Barnes, S., Grizzle, W., Miller, D. and Zhang, H. E. (2010). A Novel Nanoparticle Drug Delivery System: The Anti-Inflammatory Activity of Curcumin Is Enhanced When Encapsulated in Exosomes. *Molecular Therapy,*18 (9), 1606–1614.

Taylor, K. and Aulton, M. (2017). *Aulton's Pharmaceutics - The Design and Manufacture of Medicines.* K. Taylor and M. Aulton (Eds). 5th ed. London: Elsevier.

Teubl, B. J., Absenger, M., Fröhlich, E., Leitinger, G., Zimmer, A. and Roblegg, E. (2013). The Oral Cavity as a Biological Barrier System: Design of an Advanced Buccal *in Vitro* Permeability Model *European Journal of Pharmaceutics and Biopharmaceutics,* 84 (2), 386–393.

Tian, Y., Li, S., Song, J., Ji, T., Zhu, M., Anderson, M. J.,Wei, J. and Nie, G. (2014). A Doxorubicin Delivery Platform Using Engineered Natural Membrane Vesicle Exosomes for Targeted Tumor Therapy. *Biomaterials,* 35 (7), 2383–2390.

Tiwana, M. S., Wu, J., Hay, J., Wong, F., Cheung, W. and Olson, R. A. (2014). 25 Year Survival Outcomes for Squamous Cell Carcinomas of the Head and Neck: Population-Based Outcomes from a Canadian Province. *Oral Oncology* 50 (7), 651–656.

Unterweger, H., Subatzus, D., Tietze, R., Janko, C., Poettler, M., Stiegelschmitt, A., Schuster, M., Maake, C., Boccaccini, A. R. and Alexiou, C. (2015). Hypericin-bearing magnetic iron oxide nanoparticles for selective drug delivery in photodynamic therapy. *Int. J. Nanomed.* 10, 6985–6996.

Vasisht, N., Finn, A. (2011). *Multidirectional mucosal delivery devices and methods of use.* US0189259A1.

Velloso, N. V., Muehlmann, L. A., Longo, J. P. F., da Silva, J. R, Zancanela, D. C., Tedesco, A. C. and Azevedo, R. B. (2012). Aluminum-Phthalocyanine Chloride-Based Photodynamic Therapy Inhibits

PI3K/Akt/Mtorpathway In Oral Squamous Cell Carcinoma Cells *In Vitro*. *Chemotherapy: Open Access* 01 (05).

Wang, B., Wang, J. H., Liu, Q., Huang, H., Chen, M., Li, K., Li, C., Yu, X. F. and Chu, P. K. (2014). Rose-Bengal-Conjugated Gold Nanorods for *In vivo* Photodynamic and Photothermal Oral Cancer Therapies. *Biomaterials,* 35 (6), 1954–1966.

Wang, D., Xu, X., Zhang, K., Sun, B., Wang, L., Meng, L., Liu, Q., Zheng, C., Yang, B. and Sun, H. (2018). Codelivery of doxorubicin and MDR1-siRNA by mesoporous silica nanoparticles-polymerpolyethylenimine to improve oral squamous carcinoma treatment. *Int. J. Nanomed.* 13, 187–198.

Wang, H, Zhao, P., Liang, X., et al. (2010). Folate-PEG coated cationic modified chitosan – cholesterol liposomes for tumor-targeted drug delivery. *Biomaterials*. 31(14), 4129–4138.

Wang, W., Narain, R. and Zeng, H. (2020) Hydrogels (pp. 203-244). In: Narain R (Ed.), *Polymers science and Nanotechnology: Fundamentals and applications.* Chapter 10, Elsevier.

Wang, Z. Q., Liu, K., Huo, Z. J., Li, X. C., Wang, M., Liu, P., Pang, B. and Wang, X. J. (2015). A Cell-Targeted Chemotherapeutic Nanomedicine Strategy for Oral Squamous Cell Carcinoma Therapy. *Journal of Nanobiotechnology,* 13 (1), 1–10.

Wang, Z., Leung, M. H. M., Kee, T. W. and English, D. S. (2010). The Role of Charge in the Surfactant-Assisted Stabilization of the Natural Product Curcumin. *Langmuir,* 26 (8), 5520–5526.

Whitehead, K., Karr, N., Arora, A. and Mitragotri, S. (2012). *Oral drug devices and drug formulations.* US0045504A1.

Whittle, B. and Guy, G. (2011). *Mucoadhesive pharmaceutical formulations.* EP2298284A2.

Wu, Y. N., Yang, L. X., Shi, X. Y., Li, I. C., Biazik, I. C., Ratinac, K. R., Chen, D. H., Thordarson, P., Shieh, D. B. and Braet, F. (2011). The Selective Growth Inhibition of Oral Cancer by Iron Core-Gold Shell Nanoparticles through Mitochondria-Mediated Autophagy. *Biomaterials,* 32 (20), 4565–4573.

Yang, G., Liu, J., Wu, Y., Feng, L. and Liu Z. (2016). Near-infrared-light responsive nanoscale drug delivery systems for cancer treatment. *Coord Chem Rev*. 320-1, 100-117.

Yu, D., Wang, A., Huang, H. and Chen, Y. (2008). PEG-PBLG nanoparticle-mediated HSV-TK/GCV gene therapy for oral squamous cell carcinoma. *Nanomedicine* (Lond). 3(6), 813–821.

Zerbe, H. G., Paiement, N. (2011). *Oral mucoadhesive dosage form.* US0028431A1.

Zhang, H., Zhang, J. and Streisand J. B. (2002). Oral Mucosal Drug Delivery: Clinical Pharmacokinetics and Therapeutic Applications. *Clinical Pharmacokinetics*, 41, 661–680.

Zhao, H., Feng, H., Liu, D., Liu, J., Ji, N., Chen, F., Luo, X., et al. (2015). Self-Assembling Monomeric Nucleoside Molecular Nanoparticles Loaded with 5-FU Enhancing Therapeutic Efficacy against Oral Cancer. *ACS Nano,* 9 (10), 9638–9651.

In: Oral Squamous Cell Carcinoma
Editor: Matthew Rabin
ISBN: 978-1-53619-895-9

Chapter 3

UNRAVELING THE TARGETS OF CANCER STEM CELLS IN ORAL SQUAMOUS CELL CARCINOMA

Anjali P. Patni, Mansi Sehgal, Vaishvi Agrawal and Arikketh Devi*
Cancer Biology and Stem Cell Biology Lab,
Department of Genetic Engineering,
SRM Institute of Science and Technology, Kattankulathur,
Kanchipuram District, Tamil Nadu

ABSTRACT

Recurrence of tumors despite chemotherapy represents a profound medical condition with cancer of the oral cavity. Cancer stem cells (CSCs) have been recognized to orchestrate metastasis and facilitate tumor development in oral squamous cell carcinoma *via* the capability of self-renewal and proliferation to generate downstream progenitor cells and cancer cells. This chapter aims to highlight a detailed critical review of

* Corresponding Author's E-mail: devia@srmist.edu.in.

previous literature on putative cancer stem cell pathways for oral carcinoma and draw interest in targeting the most common cancer stem cell markers as a therapeutic regimen for oral cancer preneoplastic tumors, metastasis, and treatment progression. Thus, targeting cancer stem cells may help overcome the tumor spread and therapeutic resistance by reversing the epithelial and EMT (epithelial-to-mesenchymal transition) subpopulations shifts.

Keywords: drug resistance, signaling pathway, crosstalk, therapeutics

INTRODUCTION

Undifferentiated cells capable of self-renewing and differentiating into a vast range of distinct mature descendants are attributed as stem cells. Stem cells multiply quickly and successfully help heal tissues after injuries (Blanpain and Fuchs 2014). Given their unique regenerative abilities, stem cells are rare in most tissues. Hematopoietic stem cells (HSCs) isolated from humans and mice are the most extensively studied somatic stem cells. The term "stem cells" was coined to describe the normal tissue proliferative activity, notably the hematopoietic tissues, with constant cell replacement. In 1958, studies conducted by Hewitt confirmed the existence of cancer stem cells (CSCs) in acute myeloid leukemia before Till and McCulloch proved the origin of hematopoietic stem cells in 1961 (Hewitt 1958). Somatic stem cells and cancer cells have been compared for a long time. Cancer stem cells are labeled after normal stem cells since they possess a similar potential to self-renew and differentiate into various cell types and differ in faulty niche regulation, which causes them to differentiate and form tumors, that can spread rapidly to distant locations (Reya et al. 2001). Research has shown that only a subset of cancer cells in solid tumors can restore secondary tumors after transplantation into immunodeficient mice (Pardal, Clarke, and Morrison 2003) (Nguyen et al. 2012) (Shackleton et al. 2009). Besides, CSCs offer a plethora of distinctive properties that distinguish them from the majority of tumor cells besides self-renew and differentiation. Although CSCs were initially identified in leukemia, they have also been demonstrated in many solid tumors, such as breast, prostate, brain, colon, pancreas, and oral (cancer of oral cavity and oropharynx, along with other parts of the head and neck) cancers. In addition, CSCs have been shown to tolerate conventional cancer therapy, resulting in drug resistance and recurrence (Naik et al. 2016), and therefore eliminating CSCs in oral cancer tumors may be an effective intervention to treat oral cancer. Significant attempts have been made to investigate the signaling pathways influencing CSCs growth and self-renewal and the advancement of CSC-targeting regimens. This chapter highlights the implications of the cancer stem cells on the pathogenesis and treatment of Oral Squamous Cell Carcinoma (OSCC).

Cancer Progression in Oral Squamous Cell Carcinoma (OSCC)

Almost all tumors are heterogeneous, exhibiting distinct markers and generating several distinct and proliferative cells while primarily arising out of a single mutating cell (Melo et al. 2013). A host of solid tumors such as breast cancer, brain tumor, prostate cancer, colon cancer, and melanoma have been shown to contain cancer stem cells. Oral squamous cell carcinoma (OSCC), including head and neck squamous cell carcinoma (HNSCC) is one of the most common oral cancer in developing nations, with an elevated morbidity and mortality rate (Yj et al. 2004), (M, S, and M 2005). Any primary or metastatic lesion in oral cancer progression may contribute to malignant neoplasm from a distant or neighboring tumor site that may impact various tissues in the oral cavity. The potential risk factor for oral cancer progression includes tobacco associated oral carcinogens, alcohol intake, inadequate hygienic health, poor nutrition due to low socioeconomic conditions, and recurrent viral infections (Gillison et al. 2000). Furthermore, lineage-tracing studies reportedly demonstrated the prevalence of CSCs in the various forms of primary solid tumors, including OSCC tumors (Chiou et al. 2008, 4). Like several solid tumors, OSCC represents a wide population of cancer cells (Mehrotra and Yadav 2006) harboring cancer stem cells exhibiting characteristic features such as self-renewal, differentiation, elevated levels of stemness, tumorigenicity, spheroid growth and EMT genes (Major, Pitty, and Farah 2013).

In 2007, Prince et al. initially carried out the isolation of CSCs in HNSCC, where the group identified a subset of HNSCC cells with high CD44 expression and stem cell-like properties (Prince et al. 2007). When these CD44+ cells were injected into immunosuppressed mice, they were shown to be tumorigenic. Head and neck CSCs reside in the invasive perivascular niche, where endothelial cell signaling events initiate the survival and self-renewal of these stem cells (S. Krishnamurthy and Nör 2012).

To regulate their self-renewal ability and to keep their undifferentiated state under control, CSCs need a specific microenvironment. This specific tumor microenvironment includes stromal cells, CSCs, cytokines networks, endothelial cells and immune cells, adipocytes, secreted growth factors and carcinoma-associated fibroblasts (CAFs). Several CAF-expressed proteins were recently recognized to maintain the cancer stem cell properties in HNSCC (Bello et al. 2011). Stromal cells within the tumor niche also secretes several factors which regulate the properties of CSCs such as self-renewal. In CSCs, the hypoxic micro-environment is more preferred whereas the normal stem cells support the glycolytic micro-environment to regulate homeostasis. Hypoxia allows CSCs to sustain their undifferentiated state by accumulating genetic and epigenetic insults overtime to promote self-renewal. Both stem and non-stem cell populations gain advantage from hypoxia for self-renewal. Hypoxia triggers an elevated expression of Oct-4, Nanog, and c-Myc, which leads to the formation of spheroids, a stem cell trait. Hypoxia-inducible factors (HIFs) such as HIF1 and HIF2 serve a significant function in cancer progression and are linked to a poor cancer prognosis and also regulates cancer stem cell function by triggering Oct-4 expression. Hypoxia has been attributed as one of the main causative factor of malignant tumors of the head and neck and is also a major contributor to HNSCC resistance to chemotherapy. Accordingly, targeting hypoxic CSC niches may be a promising approach for CSCs destruction in OSCC. On the other hand, hypoxia slows cellular proliferation and, *via* HIF1, facilitates the

Warburg effect. The Warburg effect is characterized by elevated glucose intake that facilitates more lactate production triggering altered epigenetic and proliferative changes, metastasis, and drug resistance in cancer stem cells (Warburg 1956), (Stern et al. 2002), (Vander Heiden, Cantley, and Thompson 2009). The expansion of the tumor micro-environment aided by the Warburg effect may benefit the growth, survival, and invasion of cancer cells. Furthermore, Sakakura et al. elucidated the association between autophagy and immunological phenomena in the tumor microenvironment, inferring that autophagy may actively assemble immune cells, thereby elevating the tumor antigenicity towards malignant potential in oral cancer patients (Sakakura et al. 2015).

Autophagy is a crucial process regulated by a stress signaling pathway that stimulates the destruction of the damaged intracellular components to restore cellular homeostasis (Glick, Barth, and Macleod 2010). A study has recently demonstrated that autophagy is critical for aiding the phenotypic alteration in OSCC cells *via* triggering the crosstalk between carcinoma, fibroblasts, and immune cells to sustain the tumor microenvironment (Peña-Oyarzún et al. 2020). Various studies have also established the role of chemokines that may prevent autophagy in OSCC cells (Wu et al. 2011) (Min et al. 2015) (F. Lin et al. 2018). However, the precise function of autophagy in tumor development of cancer stem cells still remains uncertain. Therefore, conclusive evidences of the association between autophagy and oral cancer resistance mediated by CSCs warrants further investigation.

MECHANISMS FOR DRUG RESISTANCE IN ORAL CSCS

Surgery, radiation, and chemotherapy are the primarily established effective treatments for oral cancer. Several studies reported that individuals with recurrent oral cancer frequently develop resistance towards chemo and radiotherapy due to the presence of cancer stem cells (CSCs) (Varun, Jayanthi, and Ramani 2020). Traditional chemotherapeutic drugs are efficient in tumor debulking; nevertheless, it is hypothesized that the CSCs gradually regenerate, evade traditional therapies, and rebuild tumors locally or at remote locations over time. Minimal drug aggregation, alterations in the drug target, diminished apoptosis, and enhanced DNA damage repair are all drug resistance mechanisms in many cancers, including oral cancer. A major challenge in oncology is drug resistance that may be inherited or acquired. Dick et al. first demonstrated that CSCs (leukemic stem cells; LSCs) expressed identical genes to HSCs by utilizing a series of transplantation assays and transcriptional profiling assays (Bonnet and Dick 1997). The numerous factors that favor the expansion of CSCs consist of genetic mutations, clonal heterogeneity (Shackleton et al. 2009), tumor microenvironment (Vermeulen et al. 2010), and the survival of cancer cell sub-population with prolonged renewal potential. In the last several decades, increased multi-drug resistance to several clinically approved therapeutic agents has been a significant barrier to the effective eradication of oral cancer stem cells (da Silva et al. 2012). Cells with stem-cell-like characteristics in the basal epithelial lamina at the lesion site have been correlated to drug resistance and secondary tumor appearance in HNSCC (Q. Zhang et al. 2010). The theory on CSCs is based on understanding the dynamic evolution, phenotypic variability, and distinct epigenetic shifts (Nguyen et al. 2012). A study has demonstrated that HNSCC cells that developed resistance to Afatinib drug expressed higher levels of the stemness markers, implying that stemness may also play a role in this resistance process (Schulz et al. 2016). CSCs have various biological properties, including resistance to therapy and the ability to avoid cell death, which distinguishes them from non-CSCs (Cruz et al. 2017).

Histone deacetylases (HDACs), a well-known chromatin regulator, are dysregulated across several tumors, rendering them a potential cancer therapeutic target (Barneda-Zahonero and Parra 2012). A study demonstrated the significant function of HDACs in the modulation of EMT, stemness properties and HNSCC tolerance to chemotherapy (Giudice et al. 2013). Furthermore, it is stated that Snail (Zinc finger protein SNAI1) transcription factor recruits HDACs to facilitate E-cadherin promoter repression, thus eliciting EMT and chemoresistance in the CSCs population (Skrzypek and Majka 2020).

Drug-resistant CSCs are present primarily in the hypoxic niches and often have mitochondrial DNA mutations since they mainly depend upon glycolysis for cell survival. In other words, fewer mitochondria lead to reduced citrate intake, cytotoxicity and tolerance to cytotoxic drugs (Icard, Poulain, and Lincet 2012) (Icard et al. 2018). The hypoxic microenvironment has been shown to impose selective pressure on the development of aggressive tumors with improved metastatic capacity, decreased apoptosis, and enhanced chemoresistance in various cancers (Q. Lin and Yun 2010) (Tong, Tong, and Liu 2018). Li et al. reported that drugs including 5-FU, cisplatin, adriamycin, paclitaxel, and gemcitabine are transported more efficiently under a hypoxic environment, contributing to fewer intracellular aggregation and laryngeal carcinoma cytotoxicity (D. W. Li et al. 2013). Besides, identifying CSC drug resistance mechanisms is critical for cancer therapy and recurrence prevention in OSCC.

ORAL CANCER STEM CELL MARKERS

For the principles of stem-cell biology to apply to tumorigenesis, cancers would have to be organized hierarchically into clonally derived populations of cells with different proliferative potentials — just like cells within normal tissues.

Decades ago, it was found that when cancer cells of many different types were assayed for their proliferative potential in various *in vitro* or *in vivo* assays, only a small minority of cells were able to proliferate extensively. This gave rise to the hypothesis that malignant tumors are comprised of both cancer stem cells, which have great proliferative potential, as well as more differentiated cancer cells, with limited proliferative potential.

Table 1. CSCs markers in Oral squamous cell carcinoma

Sr. no.	Gene name	Protein name	Expression pattern in normal cells	Expression pattern in cancer stem cells	Tumorigenic property	References
1	SOX2	SRY Sex Determining Region Y-Box2	SOX2 maintains stemness and pluripotency of normal stem cells by regulating gene transcription.	oral squamous cell carcinoma (OSCC)	SOX2 regulates stemness and upregulates CSC-related gene expression SOX2 promote invasiveness and self-renewal property, and one of the members of cancer stemness related genes.	(Yoshihama et al. 2016)
2	ALDH1	Aldehyde dehydrogenase 1	Mainly plays role in the conversion of retinaldehyde to retinoic acid	head and neck squamous cell carcinoma (HNSCC)	Cells display radioresistance Displays a shift in epithelial-mesenchymal transition (EMT) endogenously co-expressed Snail protein	(Y. C. Chen et al. 2009)
3	CD133	Prominin 1, PROM1	CD133 mainly plays role in the cellular proliferation of human embryonic stem cells and developing tissues	Mainly in solid tumors	CD133 positive cells are located in the hypoxic regions of the tumor mass Cells display higher radio-/chemo-resistance	(Grosse-Gehling et al. 2013)
4	CD24	human cell surface antigen CD24 is a sialoglycoprotein	CD24 is a cell adhesion molecule that mediates growth and differentiation signal of B cells	oral squamous cell carcinoma (OSCC)	A small subgroup of CSCs expressing CD24 contributes to the onset, maintenance, and extension of tumor growth, as well as angiogenesis.	(Ghuwalewala et al. 2016) (Mirhashemi et al. 2020)
5	CD44	cell-surface glycoprotein	involved in cell–cell interactions, cell adhesion and migration.	oral squamous cell carcinoma (OSCC)	Mainly interferes with intercellular binding, migration, and angiogenesis of cancer cells	(Ghuwalewala et al. 2016)
6	CD47	Integrin-associated signal transducer or protein (IAST or IAP)	It is an antigenic surface determinant protein that provides a "self" or "do not eat" signal by interacting with the signal regulatory protein alpha (SIRPα) on immune cells to suppress or inhibit macrophage phagocytosis	Oral squamous cell carcinoma (OSCC)	CD47 promotes orosphere formation, colony formation, and reduced radiosensitivity in OSCC *via* upregulation of CD47-CSCs-EMT signaling loop.	(Pai et al. 2019)

Sr. no.	Gene name	Protein name	Expression pattern in normal cells	Expression pattern in cancer stem cells	Tumorigenic property	References
7	ITGA7	Integrin α7	Play role in cell-cell and cell-matrix interactions, cell migration, morphologic development, and differentiation	tongue squamous cell carcinoma (TSCC)	upregulated in the tumor tissues compared with the paired adjacent tissues Serve as a potential marker for CSCs	(Lv, Yang, and Yang 2020)
8	BMI1	BMI1 protooncogene, polycomb ring finger protein	Plays a crucial role in regulating the proliferative activity of normal stem and progenitor cells.	tongue squamous cell carcinoma (TSCC)	Mediates the migration and invasion of TSCC mediated *via* C-myc-Bmi1-SOD2 pathway that trigger metastasis	(He et al. 2015)
9	CMTM6	CKLF-like MARVEL transmembrane domain-containing 6	Play a key role in secretory proteins and plays multiple roles in physiological and pathological processes	Oral squamous cell carcinoma (OSCC)	Highly expresses in cancer tissues and is associated with OSCC metastasis and patient prognosis CMTM6 crosstalk with NRP1 in both OSCC tissues and cell lines promote cell migration and invasion	(L. Chen et al. 2020) (Zheng et al. 2020, 1)
10	KLF4	KRUPPEL-LIKE FACTOR 4	Mainly involved in tissue development, differentiation and maintenance of homeostasis	Oral squamous cell carcinoma (OSCC)	Induces the CSCs phenotype in the skin and in fibroblasts. KLF4 can function as a transforming oncogene *in vitro*,	(Roy et al. 2019)
11	Cripto 1/ TDGF1	Cripto-1 growth factor/ Teratocarcinoma-derived growth factor 1	membrane-bound protein that plays an essential role in embryonic development and tumor growth.	Oral squamous cell carcinoma (OSCC)	play a role in the malignant transformation of oral mucosa, involved in the tumorigenesis and progression of OSCC by enhancing tumor cell growth and motility.	(Yoon et al. 2011)

Cancer stem cells promote tumor development by expressing unique cell surface markers that may trigger tumor relapse even after cancer-therapy (Y. Li et al. 2015). CSCs encode several genes in common with early ESCs (Ben-Porath et al. 2008), particularly OCT4, NANOG, and SOX2 that are also overexpressed in human malignancies and it could be attributed to tumorigenicity, tumor metastasis, and distant recurrence after chemoradiotherapy. Stem cell markers for identifying and differentiating the various stages of oral cancers have been applied recently. Studies have shown significant associations between the expression of both OCT4 and NANOG that may be effective prognostic markers in patients with oral squamous cell carcinoma. OCT4, the most important pluripotent factor, has been detected to be up-regulated in several human cancers, including OSCC (Chiou et al. 2008).

Studies have demonstrated that $CD24^{+}/CD44^{+}$ populations marked elevated EMT properties along with enhanced expression of drug transporters, thereby inducing prolonged chemoresistance in patients with oral cancer stem cells (Ghuwalewala et al. 2016) (Table 1).

Diagnostic Approaches in the Determination of CSCs in OSCC

OSCC tissue possesses a structural composition identical to the origin tissue inclusive to that of CSCs. Oral CSCs diagnosis can be anticipated by the tumor stage and size. (Deepthi Sogasu, Devaraj Ezhilarasan, and Smiline Girija AS 2020). However, various methods can be applied to perform differential characterizations of the CSCs, including spherical formation tests (O'Brien, Kreso, and Jamieson 2010), flow cytometric surface marker sorting, Xenograft Formation Assay (Calvet, André, and Mir 2014), Orosphere Assay (Sudha Krishnamurthy and Nör 2013), Aldefluor assay, and the Hoechst side population (SP) technique (Shimoda, Ota, and Okada 2018) (Bhutia et al. 2019).

In 2008, Stanford University performed a feasibility analysis to examine whether CSCs obtained from surgical tissue biopsies of head and neck cancers (NCT00610415) were adequately quantified by flow cytometry.

Some of the methods include:

- Hoechst Dye Method - A characteristic flow cytometric profile with dye-excluding cells distinct from the main cell population is referred to as side population (SP) cells. The identification of CSC is done with SPs where Hoechst 33342 is eliminated, which is a fluorescent DNA binding dye and it generally binds to A-T rich regions. They express high levels of ABC transporters. When ABCB5 expression is high it is associated with the progression of OSCC making it a probable prognostic factor. CSCs were identified in OSCC-derived side population cells and targeting CD133 sensitized CSCs to chemotherapies (C.-C. Yu et al. 2016).
- Sphere Formation Assay - It is an *in vitro* method that is extensively accepted for the characterization and advancement of CSCs based on these cells' integral property of self-renewal capacity. Lim et al. identified CSCs characteristics in squamospheres resulting from OSCCs, implying that the animal cancer model could be used to investigate CSC in human oral cancers in the future (Lim et al. 2011). The sphere formation and xenograft growth can be suppressed by Honokiol, a potential oral cancer treatment drug where it suppresses the growth of oral CSCs both *in vitro* and *in vivo* (Huang et al. 2016). This proposes its potency as an integrative medicine for combating oral cancer through CSCs targeting.
- Orosphere Formation assay - Sorted Side Population cells from several OSCC cell lines grew as three-dimensional spheres called orospheres. Telomeric Repeat Binding Factor-2 (TRF2) maintains genomic stability by preventing activation of the DNA damage repair pathways at the telomeric end and also maintains and assists in the formation of orosphere. Study has determined the role of curcumin in progressively reducing the self-renewal property and primary orospheres formatting ability in a dose dependent manner

in both Human Papilloma Virus (virus (HPV positive/HPV negative) Oral CSCs (Bano, Yadav, and Das 2018).

- Aldefluor Assay - It is used for the isolation of CSCs from OSCC cell lines. Aldehyde dehydrogenase 1 (ALDH1) is a CSC marker and its presence strongly indicates tumor malignancy, self-renewal of stem cells, increased invasion rate and expresses resistance to chemotherapeutic agents. It also indicates radiotherapy resistance and disease staging in OSCC. When it combines with other CSC markers like CD133 and CD44, it accelerates the isolation process of tumorigenic subpopulation which is a primary feature of CSCs in OSCC. An ALDEFLUOR bright (ALDH1br) population is found in all of the cell lines where it efficaciously produce tumor spheres than ALDH1 low cells and display escalated levels of stem cell markers including SOX2 and NANOG; thus, ALDH1br cells are likely to be enhanced by CSC population and should be suitable for analysis of Oral CSCs (Michifuri et al. 2012).

Flow cytometry using cell surface markers- Some stem cell markers have been identified for normal oral epithelium and most of them are intracellular markers which are unsuitable for flow sorting. Some of the potential markers for cytometry are β1-integrin, α6-integrin, CD71 (transferrin receptor), CD44, E-cadherin, β-catenin. In OSCC-derived cell lines, colonies with holoclone morphologies show consistently higher levels of expression of stem cell-related molecules such as β1-integrin, E-cadherin, β-catenin (Felthaus et al. 2011). CD44 has been reported as one of the most abundantly expressed marker in OSCC. Also, it has the potential of diagnosing OSCC at an early stage. It was detected in OSCC through immunohistochemistry analysis. CSCs can also be reliably detected immunohistochemically in fixed human tissues of OSCC and in all the control specimens.

Gene expression and Western Blot analyses showed that patients with recurrent OSCC have an escalated expression of CSC markers (KLF4 and OCT4) along with β-catenin in the surgical cut margin (CM) region compared with the tumor counterpart. In contrast, in non-recurrent OSCC, increased expression of KLF4, OCT4, and β-catenin were observed in the tumor region as compared with the CM region (Roy et al. 2019). Oct4 regulates the stemness of OSCC by enhancing tumor invasion, promoting tumor growth and aiding the formation of CSC like cells by encouraging de-differentiation of differentiated OSCC cells. The overexpression of Oct4 in OSCC helps in identifying the early stages of the disease and has an improved prognosis.

PUTATIVE SIGNALING PATHWAYS TRIGGERING THE CSCS PROLIFERATION IN OSCC

According to Eppert et al., CSCs are governed by core molecular pathways similar to those expressed by HSCs (Eppert et al. 2011). A variety of signaling mechanisms are currently being investigated as alternative therapies. Numerous signaling pathways have been identified that regulate the self-renewal and proliferative ability of CSCs that include Notch (Pannuti et al. 2010), Wnt/β-Catenin (Takahashi-Yanaga and Kahn 2010), and Hedgehog pathway (Takezaki et al. 2011).

The highly conserved Notch signaling pathway plays a role in regulating embryonic development, stem cell renewal, differentiation, proliferation and homeostasis. Furthermore, activated canonical and non-canonical Notch signaling pathways are prevalent in most cases of cancer metastasis. There are four Notch receptors (Notch 1, 2, 3, and 4) (Meurette and Mehlen 2018), five Notch ligands (Jagged ligands: JAG1 and JAG2 and Delta-like ligands: DLL1, DLL3, and DLL4) (Rebay et al. 1991), activators, repressors, transcription factors and downstream effectors in the Notch cascade. Activation of the Notch receptor results in the release of NICD (the Notch intracellular domain) from the plasma membrane, and its translocation into the nucleus leads to recruitment of the CSL (CBF1, Suppressor of hairless and LAG-1 domain) transcription factors to trigger the expression of the downstream Hes (Hairy enhancer of split) and Hey (Hairy enhancer of split similar to YRPW motif) family genes. The Notch signaling pathway is becoming a widely known target for CSCs elimination since it intricately associates the process of angiogenesis to the self-renewal of CSCs. Activation of the Notch pathway in several human cancers generally facilitates survival, self-renewal induces metastasis and impedes apoptosis in CSCs (Harrison et al. 2010). Lee et al. demonstrated that Notch1 inhibition slows tumorigenesis and decreases the incidence of self-renewal of HNSCC in xenografts (Sang H. Lee et al. 2016). Inhibition of Notch signaling found in HNSCC cell lines, thus prevents the development of primary spheres. Similarly, Notch1 inhibition by a gamma-secretase inhibitor (DAPT) can suppress tumorigenesis and CSC self-renewal in HNSCC (Zhao et al. 2016). The regulatory activation of the NICD facilitated the self-renewal ability of HNSCC cells, and the expression of stem cell markers was increased as a result. The perturbation of the NOTCH pathway shows a reduction in HNSCC ability to migrate and the subsequent formation of cancer stem-like features and highlights their need for the progression. Lee et al. determined the role of the proinflammatory cytokine, TNFα (tumor necrosis factor α), in improving self-renewal capability and tumorigenicity correlated with the activation of the Notch signaling pathway wherein Notch1–Hes1 axis regulates oral CSCs self-renewal. In TNFα-induced OSCC, Hes1 is a target of activated Notch1, and its inactivation suppresses the self-renewal potential (Sung Hee Lee et al. 2012). Hence. by regulating Slug and Twist's expression, Notch1 stimulates TNFα-induced OSCC invasiveness *via* the activation of the Notch-Hes1 pathway and encourages sphere-forming capability, stemness-related gene expression, chemo-radio-resistance, and tumorigenicity in oral cancer cells. These findings are all in conjunction with studies that indicate that Notch signaling is needed for stem cell-like features in many forms of cancer. The genetic determinants of CSCs often affect tumorigenesis. These findings are in consistent with previous reports, which suggest that Notch signaling is needed for stem cell-like characteristics in various types of OSCC tumors.

The Wnt signaling pathway (canonical and non-canonical Wnt signaling pathway) is a conserved developmental pathway that governs embryogenesis, homeostasis, fate determination, stem cell renewal, and differentiation (J. Wang, Sinha, and Wynshaw-Boris 2012) (Nusse and

Clevers 2017). The canonical Wnt/β-catenin signaling pathway is triggered by Wnt ligands binding to Frizzled (Fzd) and its co-receptor, LRP 5/6 (lipoprotein receptor-related protein 5 or 6), which then dissociates the β-catenin degradation complex and allows translocation of β-catenin into the nucleus to promote transcription of downstream targets via binding to the N-terminal of TCF/LEF (T-cell factor/lymphoid enhancing factor) transcription factors (Niehrs 2012). The abnormal expression of β-catenin has been suggested to be essential in the development and progression of OSCC (Z. Yu et al. 2005). Intriguingly, patients with primary OSCC tumors displayed a lower survival rate with elevated nuclear β-catenin expression (Pukkila et al. 2001). Further, the immunohistochemical analysis found that metastatic lymph node samples of OSCC patients had decreased E-cadherin and β-catenin expression (Tanaka et al. 2003). In addition, the activation of the Wnt pathway is essential in the proliferation of CSC-like cells in OSCC cells (Felthaus et al. 2011). Furthermore, an antagonist of the Wnt pathway, secreted frizzled-related protein 4 (sFRP4), was reported to lower the expression of stemness markers CD44, ALDH, drug resistance markers ABCG2 and ABCC4, and stimulate cell death induced by cisplatin (Sudha Warrier et al. 2013). Besides, sFRP4 therapy can reverse HNSCC EMT as demonstrated by the downregulation of Twist, Snail, and N-cadherin mesenchymal markers subsequently by restoration of E-cadherin epithelial marker, indicating the crucial function of Wnt/b-catenin signaling in the CSCs maintenance and proliferation (S. Warrier et al. 2014). Likewise, activation of the Wnt signaling pathway in HNSCC improved CSCs characteristics such as tumor invasion and sphere formation (Le et al. 2019). Numerous nonsteroidal anti-inflammatory drugs, such as aspirin and celecoxib, as well as phytochemicals such as epigallocatechin-3-gallate (EGCG), resveratrol, honokiol, curcumin, and others, have been reported as inhibitors of the Wnt/β-catenin signalling system in combating the development and proliferation of oral cancer stem cells (Yao et al. 2013) (Reyes et al. 2020). Similarly, HC-1, a derivative of hexachlorophene, has been shown to inhibit Wnt signaling by fostering E3 ubiquitination ligase by seven absentia homolog 1 (SIAH1)-dependent β-catenin degradation, leading to decreased CSCs populations in OSCC (Yokogi et al. 2016).

Hedgehog signaling is indispensable during embryogenesis, homeostasis, and animal development (Ingham and McMahon 2001). The Hedgehog protein interaction with its receptor, Ptch1 (Patched-1), induces the transcription factor Gli (Glioma-related oncogene homolog 1) to become activated triggering the activation of downstream target genes such as Ptch and Gli (Bale 2002). The function of the Shh pathway in several animal models has been well considered amongst these three types of Hedgehog genes, Sonic Hedgehog (Shh), Desert Hedgehog (Dhh), and Indian Hedgehog (Ihh) (Varjosalo and Taipale 2007). Hedgehog signaling plays a role in the induction and progression of a variety of cancers (Qijin Xu et al. 2008). Overexpression of the Hedgehog pathway is critical in the OSCC progression, and SHH signal activation is correlated with a poor prognosis. Similarly, suppression the SHH signaling pathway has shown to prevent tumor growth and angiogenesis in HNSCC in a consistent manner (Kuroda et al. 2017). In addition, The Hedgehog signaling pathway transcriptionally regulates the expression of EMT-specific markers Snail and Twist1, which retains CSC properties, displays the chemoresistant phenotype, and eventually regulates the expression of ATP-binding cassette transporters (ABC transporters) that facilitate drug resistance in OSCC (Kong et al. 2015).

The Janus kinase (JAK) signal transducer and activator of the transcription (STAT) pathway is another essential target pathway in oral cancer (Lai and Johnson 2010). Several interferons, cytokines, and growth factors stimulate the JAK/STAT (Janus kinase, signal transducer and activator of transcription protein) signaling pathway, which is involved in tumor signaling. Seven STAT family members have been described in mammals till date. Cytokines or growth factors facilitate STAT binding and phosphorylation by rendering extracellular stimulation for activating JAK by transphosphorylation. The transiently activated STATs dimerize in the nucleus to serve as transcription factors, regulating gene expression in cell growth, production, differentiation, inflammation and survival processes. The dimeric STAT proteins are then inactivated and returned to the cytoplasm *via* tyrosine dephosphorylation. Several studies have reported that STAT3 is constitutively expressed in a host of solid human tumors, including head and neck cancers (Lai and Johnson 2010). Upregulation of STAT3 target genes such as Bcl-2 (B-cell lymphoma 2), c-myc (cellular-myelocytomatosis), cyclin D1, and VEGF (Vascular endothelial growth factor) *via* constitutive activation of STAT3 affects cancer cell growth and directs tumor progression. Furthermore, overexpression of STAT3 has been linked to cisplatin resistance in HNSCC (Gu et al. 2010). Likewise, elevated STAT3 phosphorylation promotes Cetuximab resistance in the HNSCC patient tumors (Sen et al. 2012) (Willey et al. 2019). Similarly, the role of Honokiol, a phytochemical compound, has also been demonstrated by Huang et al. in preventing sphere formation and xenograft development in oral CSC-like cells linked to apoptosis activation, inactivation of angiogenesis as well as the survival/proliferation-promoting JAK2/STAT3 signaling pathway (Huang et al. 2016). Extensive attempts have also been made to target STAT3 signaling with new therapeutic strategies that can trigger apoptosis and chemotherapy favoring tumor-sensitization.

A significant role of the protein kinase B (AKT)/ mammalian target of the rapamycin (mTOR) pathway has been highlighted in the development of OSCC (Harsha et al. 2020). The cancer genome atlas (TCGA) analysis reported that a higher proportion of HNSCC cases had an abnormal level of AKT/mTOR signaling pathway (Vander Broek et al. 2015). Phosphoinositide 3-kinase (PI3K), AKT, and mTOR proteins are the primary regulators of this pathway. The AKT/mTOR pathway is activated by the receptor tyrosine kinases (RTKs) and cytokine receptors. Phosphorylated tyrosine residues serve as binding sites for PI3K translocation to the nuclear membrane, allowing it to participate in the transduction of a variety of extracellular matrix molecules and cytokines. AKT acts as the vital molecule downstream of the PI3K signaling pathway, while mTOR functions downstream of AKT. Kuo et al. demonstrated the function of Salinomycin, a monocarboxylic polyether antibiotic, in triggering cell death and differentiation in HNSCC cancer stem cells through EMT and AKT signalling activation (Kuo et al. 2012).

Epidermal Growth Factor Receptor (EGFR) is usually expressed at high levels in various types of cancer and is therefore significantly related to tumor proliferation and unfavorable clinical prognosis (S. J. Wang and

Bourguignon 2006). EGFR is a tyrosine kinase receptor protein that performs an essential function in the survival, progression, and differentiation of epithelial tumor cells (carcinoma) (Talukdar et al. 2020). The EGFR signaling pathway activation has been reported to be related to the cancer cell phenotype, apoptosis suppression, defined angiogenesis, and metastasis, respectively. EGFR signaling is predominantly expressed in HNSCCs, regulating a distinct population that possesses stem cell-like properties (J. S. Chen et al. 2006). Similarly, one of the known hallmarks of metastatic HNSCC is over-expressed EGFR (Ryott et al. 2009). It is further essential to point out that CSC cells also express the CD44 cell surface marker associated with EGFR, enhancing the HNSCC tumorigenicity (Perez et al. 2013). A recent study demonstrated that EGFR signaling contributes to enhancing HNSCC stemness and progression by decreasing SOX2 autophagic deterioration and growing its stability; therefore, targeting EGFR in conjunction with traditional chemotherapy could be a promising approach to treat HNSCC via CSC elimination (X.-X. Lv et al. 2020, 2).

Numerous pathways do not function discretely but engage as a biological network (crosstalk) in the growth and homeostasis with several other pathways. For instance, Nair et al. demonstrated that mutations in the EGFR extracellular domain would result in (EGF)-independent signaling, resulting in persistent AKT signaling and tolerance to cetuximab (Nair et al. 2020). Moreover, the association of Notch with the Wnt and Hedgehog signaling pathways has uncovered new knowledge regarding CSCs survival and function in OSCC (Patni et al. 2021).

miRNAs (MicroRNAs, small non-coding molecules) regulate gene expression at the post-transcriptional stage and are prevalent in almost all cellular processes. miRNAs are often implicated in multiple cancer pathogenesis, including oral squamous cell carcinoma. Similarly, lncRNAs (long non-coding RNA) molecules are reported to regulate cellular processes and have been implicated in cancer drug resistance (Kolenda et al. 2017). Studies have identified that miRNAs and lncRNAs play a significant function in CSCs regulation (Asadzadeh et al. 2019) (Yan and Bu 2018).

CSCs formation can be hindered by targeting a potential tumor suppressor or by blocking/impairing the molecules of signaling pathways that would work to slow down metastasis and halt recurrence.

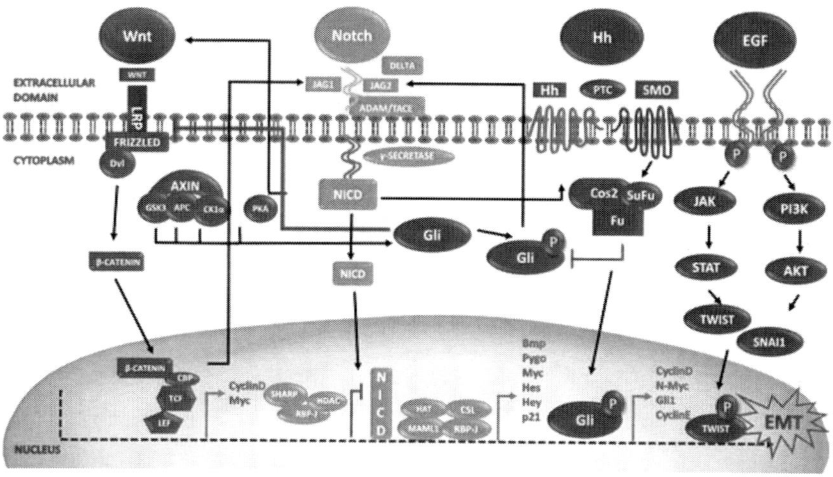

Figure 1. Putative signaling pathways in Oral cancer stem cells).

EPITHELIAL TO MESENCHYMAL TRANSITION (EMT) AND ORAL CANCER STEM CELLS

EMT (increase in mesenchymal markers and decline in the epithelial markers) is a vital aspect in the progress of embryogenesis and wound healing processes, allowing epithelial cells to disintegrate cell to cell and cell to matrix contacts that facilitate their movement to other locations in the body. EMT favors the development of metastasis in pathologic conditions such as wound healing and epithelial cancers (Barriere et al. 2015). The evolutionarily conserved process of EMT is classified into 3 distinct types: EMT-1 (normal embryogenesis), EMT-2 (tissue regeneration and wound healing), and EMT-3 (cancer progression) (Kalluri and Weinberg 2009). CSCs can execute EMT, thus enabling the genetic factors involved, including cell contact break down and migration, which permits tumor cell metastasis (Roche 2018).

As cancer cells undergo EMT, they fail their epithelial characteristics and achieve mesenchymal features such as fibroblast-like morphology, altered gene expression patterns, and enhanced motility (Scheel and Weinberg 2012). Furthermore, metastasis is often related to self-renewal and is a distinctive mark of CSCs. Through the suppression of E-cadherin, the importance of EMT in promoting CSCs properties was explicitly demonstrated by the rise in the expression of pluripotency genes, including Oct4 and Nanog (van de Stolpe 2013). In local relapse and lymph node metastasis, EMT performs a critical role and is correlated with a high mortality rate in OSCC patients. Thierauf et al. initially demonstrated the clinical significance of a mesenchymal-like phenotype of both the Kallikrein-related peptidase 6 (KLK6) and the pluripotency-associated transcription factor sex-determining region Y-box 2 (SOX2) in head and neck cancer patients (Thierauf, Veit, and Hess 2017).

The epithelial to mesenchymal transition (EMT) of $ALDH^+$ $CD44^+$ CSCs in HNSCC is encouraged by endothelial cells *via* secreting epidermal growth factors (EGFs) (Z. Zhang et al. 2014). Previous studies have shown that Twist-related protein 1 (TWIST1) is a significant modulator of EMT (Peng et al. 2015). A study has shown the role of TWIST1 that activates a Polycomb complex protein BMI-1 (Proto-Oncogene, Polycomb Ring Finger) to promote stemness and metastasis in HNSCC (Yang et al. 2010). Also, transcription factor Snail was reported to suppress E-cadherin expression and enhance HNSCC motility and invasiveness through EMT, enhancing cancer stem-like properties and cisplatin-resistance in HNSCC (Masui et al. 2014). Thus, TWIST1 should be investigated further as a possible target for overcoming acquired resistance because it has been involved in many important mechanisms that may evoke drug resistance in oral cancer stem cells (Table 2).

Table 2. Factors involved in the regulation of epithelial to mesenchymal transition in oral cancer stem cells

Sr no.	Gene name	Protein name	Expression in normal cells	Role in oral cancer stem cells	Mechanism	References
	ADAR1	Adenosine deaminases acting on RNA1	It plays a part in RNA-editing during post transcriptional modification (PTM) of mRNA transcripts by modifying the nucleotide content (adenosine to inosine *via* deamination).	The epithelial to mesenchymal transition (EMT), stemness, and malignant phenotype of OSCC cell lines are triggered by overexpression of ADAR1.	Overexpressed ADAR1 may facilitate OSCC progression by promoting the EMT and oncogenic miRNAs maturation via interaction with the Dicer protein.	(Liu et al. 2019)
	TWIST1	Twist Family Bhlh Transcription Factor 1	Twist1 protein is mainly involved in the regulation of organogenesis and development	Twist1 strongly expresses in patients with advanced OSCC, and its expression level is correlated with metastasis formation and poor survival	Elevated level of Twist1 activates the transcription of Bmi1, a chromatin modifier, and interacts with Bmi1-containing PRC1/2 to suppress E-cadherin expression; that induces EMT	(da Silva et al. 2014) (Zhu et al. 2016)
	SNAI1	Snail Family Transcriptional Repressor 1	Snail is indispensable for mesoderm formation and early embryogenesis	play a transcrip-tional and regulatory role in the invasion, metastasis and poor outcome in different type of malignancies, including HNSCC	plays an important role in regulating CSC-like properties via EMT by directly repressing epithelial markers such as E-cadherin and by upregulating mesenchymal markers	(Ota et al. 2016)
	EGF	epidermal growth factor	EGF promotes cellular proliferation, differentiation, and survival through binding to the EGFR receptor.	EGF elicits the Warburg effect that promotes EMT and cancer stem-like cell features in human oral cancer cells.	*Via* EGFR/PI3K/HIF-1 axis-driven glycolytic metabolism, EGF stimulates EMT and CSCs progression in OSCC cells.	(Xu et al. 2017)
	CCL21/CCR7	chemokine ligand 21 and C-C chemokine receptor 7	CCL21 binds to its CCR7 receptor prevents hemopoiesis and induces chemotaxis, as well as facilitates lymphocyte homing	CCR7 and CCL21 highly expresses in OSCC tissues.	The JAK2/STAT3 signaling pathway engage in CCL21/CCR7 regulated EMT and stemness of Oral cancer cells	(Y. Chen et al. 2020)

Table 2. (Continued)

Sr no.	Gene name	Protein name	Expression in normal cells	Role in oral cancer stem cells	Mechanism	References
	NRP1	NEUROPILIN 1	It has been identified as a co-receptor for multiple growth factors, including VEGF-A, FGF, HGF and others, and is expressed on epithelial cells	NRP1 promoted the EMT process through NF-κB activation	NRP1could interact with CMTM6 thus mediate cell proliferation, tumorigenesis, immune response and invasion.	(Zheng et al. 2020, 1)
	BRACHYURY	T-box transcription factor brachyury	Very essential for mesoderm formation during early development	BRACHUARY regulates the EMT) and CSC potential in human salivary and oral carcinoma cells	Synergistically interact with SOX2 SOX2 to regulate CSC and EMT (invasiveness) phenotype.	(Fernando et al. 2010) (Akimoto et al. 2018)

FUTURE THERAPEUTICS AND POSSIBLE CLINICAL IMPLICATIONS OF CSCs IN OSCC

Identifying cancer-like stem cells has been a critical challenge, particularly with a promising future targeted therapy. CSCs have been moved to the frontline of cancer treatment due to their association with tumor induction and drug resistance.

Several cell-signaling inhibitors targeting oral cancer stem cells have been developed recently, including biological agents and small molecular agents. For instance, a small LGK974 inhibitor was shown to be effective in targeting Wnt signals in several cancer models, including HNSCC. Although, no inhibitors of Wnt signals for therapeutic use have, however, been clinically permitted to date. Another promising drug namely, Rapamycin prevents cancer metabolism by selectively inhibiting mTORC1. Phase 1 and 2 clinical trial studies (NCT01195922) of HNSCC patients revealed positive results (Day et al. 2019). Rapamycin, however, had little effect in HNSCC patients when combined with another drug. Similarly, Gefitinib, a tyrosine-specific EGFR kinase inhibitor, has shown promising results in the treatment of HNSCC since it impacts CSC activity by explicitly targeting the CSCs population (X.-X. Lv et al. 2020, 2).

Lee et al. recently demonstrated the role of bisphosphonate medication, namely zoledronic acid (ZA, commercially also known as zoledronate), in targeting oral CSCs by suppressing the expression pattern of chemokine C-C motif ligand 3 (CCL3), where its signal activation elicits the CSC function in OSCC cells (Sung Hee Lee et al. 2021, 3). According to studies, the stromal microenvironment, including the CSCs niche, serve a vital function in cancer cell activity (Tang, Ang, and Pervaiz 2007), and therefore explicitly targeting the stem cell niche will disrupt the critical signaling cascade required for CSC proliferation and growth.

Conclusion

Cancer stem cells constitute a limited percentage of tumor cells that can regenerate developing tumors. Consequently, while CSC-targeting therapeutics are still in their infancy, targeting the CSC population has been a successful form of cancer treatment. While extensive research in determining the characteristics of CSCs in OSCC has been conducted where all of these studies converged on *in vitro* data, none have progressed ahead of the early stages of clinical trials. As previously reported, a deeper understanding of CSC properties and druggable goals is needed to create new strategies for targeting CSCs in OSCC. Nonetheless, the signaling pathways interact in a synchronized manner to regulate the stemness and functionality of CSCs. CSC annihilation by addressing the primary signaling mechanisms influencing the stemness and CSCs activity could ascertain a potential cancer therapeutic approach. Accordingly, for the advancement of therapies targeting CSCs in oral cancer, identifying the crosstalk among the signaling pathways is vital. Furthermore, it is crucial to recognize that precision medicine can be of great benefit in the care of patients with varying CSC management.

References

Akimoto, Naonari, Kodai Nakamura, Hiroshi Hijioka, Kenichi Kume, Yoshiaki Matsumura, and Tsuyoshi Sugiura. 2018. "Transfection of T-Box Transcription Factor BRACHYURY and SOX2 Synergistically Promote Self-Renewal and Invasive Phenotype in Oral Cancer Cells." *International Journal of Molecular Sciences* 19 (11). https://doi.org/10.3390/ijms19113620.

Asadzadeh, Zahra, Behzad Mansoori, Ali Mohammadi, Marjan Aghajani, Khalil Haji-Asgarzadeh, Elham Safarzadeh, Ahad Mokhtarzadeh, Pascal H. G. Duijf, and Behzad Baradaran. 2019. "MicroRNAs in Cancer Stem Cells: Biology, Pathways, and Therapeutic Opportunities."

Journal of Cellular Physiology 234 (7): 10002–17. https://doi.org/10.1002/jcp.27885.

Bale, Allen E. 2002. "Hedgehog Signaling and Human Disease." *Annual Review of Genomics and Human Genetics* 3: 47–65. https://doi.org/10.1146/annurev.genom.3.022502.103031.

Bano, Nasreen, Manisha Yadav, and Bhudev C. Das. 2018. "Differential Inhibitory Effects of Curcumin between HPV+ve and HPV−ve Oral Cancer Stem Cells." *Frontiers in Oncology* 8 (September). https://doi.org/10.3389/fonc.2018.00412.

Barneda-Zahonero, Bruna, and Maribel Parra. 2012. "Histone Deacetylases and Cancer." *Molecular Oncology* 6 (6): 579–89. https://doi.org/10.1016/j.molonc.2012.07.003.

Barriere, Guislaine, Pietro Fici, Giulia Gallerani, Francesco Fabbri, and Michel Rigaud. 2015. "Epithelial Mesenchymal Transition: A Double-Edged Sword." *Clinical and Translational Medicine* 4 (April). https://doi.org/10.1186/s40169-015-0055-4.

Bello, Ibrahim O., Marilena Vered, Dan Dayan, Alex Dobriyan, Ran Yahalom, Kalle Alanen, Pentti Nieminen, Saara Kantola, Esa Läärä, and Tuula Salo. 2011. "Cancer-Associated Fibroblasts, a Parameter of the Tumor Microenvironment, Overcomes Carcinoma-Associated Parameters in the Prognosis of Patients with Mobile Tongue Cancer." *Oral Oncology* 47 (1): 33–38. https://doi.org/10.1016/j.oraloncology.2010.10.013.

Ben-Porath, Ittai, Matthew W. Thomson, Vincent J. Carey, Ruping Ge, George W. Bell, Aviv Regev, and Robert A. Weinberg. 2008. "An Embryonic Stem Cell-like Gene Expression Signature in Poorly Differentiated Aggressive Human Tumors." *Nature Genetics* 40 (5): 499–507. https://doi.org/10.1038/ng.127.

Bhutia, Sujit K., Prajna P. Naik, Prakash P. Praharaj, Debasna P. Panigrahi, Chandra S. Bhol, Kewal K. Mahapatra, Sarbari Saha, and Srimanta Patra. 2019. "Identification and Characterization of Stem Cells in Oral Cancer." *Methods in Molecular Biology (Clifton, N.J.)* 2002: 129–39. https://doi.org/10.1007/7651_2018_184.

Blanpain, Cédric, and Elaine Fuchs. 2014. "Plasticity of Epithelial Stem Cells in Tissue Regeneration." *Science (New York, N.Y.)* 344 (6189): 1242281. https://doi.org/10.1126/science.1242281.

Bonnet, D., and J. E. Dick. 1997. "Human Acute Myeloid Leukemia Is Organized as a Hierarchy That Originates from a Primitive Hematopoietic Cell." *Nature Medicine* 3 (7): 730–37. https://doi.org/10.1038/nm0797-730.

Calvet, Christophe Y., Franck M. André, and Lluis M. Mir. 2014. "The Culture of Cancer Cell Lines as Tumorspheres Does Not Systematically Result in Cancer Stem Cell Enrichment." *PloS One* 9 (2): e89644. https://doi.org/10.1371/journal.pone.0089644.

Chen, Jocelyn S., Francisco S. Pardo, Jessica Wang-Rodriguez, Theresa S. Chu, Jay Patrick Lopez, Joseph Aguilera, Xabier Altuna, Robert A. Weisman, and Weg M. Ongkeko. 2006. "EGFR Regulates the Side Population in Head and Neck Squamous Cell Carcinoma." *The Laryngoscope* 116 (3): 401–6. https://doi.org/10.1097/01.mlg.0000195075.14093.fb.

Chen, Lei, Qi-Chao Yang, Yi-Cun Li, Lei-Lei Yang, Jian-Feng Liu, Hao Li, Yao Xiao, Lin-Lin Bu, Wen-Feng Zhang, and Zhi-Jun Sun. 2020. "Targeting CMTM6 Suppresses Stem Cell-Like Properties and Enhances Antitumor Immunity in Head and Neck Squamous Cell Carcinoma." *Cancer Immunology Research* 8 (2): 179–91. https://doi.org/10.1158/2326-6066.CIR-19-0394.

Chen, Yang, Zhe Shao, Erhui Jiang, Xiaocheng Zhou, Lin Wang, Hui Wang, Xinyue Luo, Qingli Chen, Ke Liu, and Zhengjun Shang. 2020. "CCL21/CCR7 Interaction Promotes EMT and Enhances the Stemness of OSCC via a JAK2/STAT3 Signaling Pathway." *Journal of Cellular Physiology* 235 (9): 5995–6009. https://doi.org/10.1002/jcp.29525.

Chen, Yu-Chih, Yi-Wei Chen, Han-Shui Hsu, Ling-Ming Tseng, Pin-I. Huang, Kai-Hsi Lu, Dow-Tien Chen, et al. 2009. "Aldehyde Dehydrogenase 1 Is a Putative Marker for Cancer Stem Cells in Head and Neck Squamous Cancer." *Biochemical and Biophysical Research Communications* 385 (3): 307–13. https://doi.org/10.1016/j.bbrc.2009.05.048.

Chiou, Shih-Hwa, Cheng-Chia Yu, Chi-Yang Huang, Shu-Chun Lin, Chung-Ji Liu, Tung-Hu Tsai, Shiu-Huey Chou, Chian-Shiu Chien, Hung-Hai Ku, and Jeng-Fan Lo. 2008. "Positive Correlations of Oct-4 and Nanog in Oral Cancer Stem-like Cells and High-Grade Oral Squamous Cell Carcinoma." *Clinical Cancer Research: An Official Journal of the American Association for Cancer Research* 14 (13): 4085–95. https://doi.org/10.1158/1078-0432.CCR-07-4404.

Cruz, Ana Filipa, Nuno Andre Fonseca, Vera Moura, Sergio Simoes, and Joao Nuno Moreira. 2017. "Targeting Cancer Stem Cells and Non-Stem Cancer Cells: The Potential of Lipid-Based Nanoparticles." *Current Pharmaceutical Design*, November. https://doi.org/10.2174/13 81612823666171115105252.

Day, Terry A., Keisuke Shirai, Paul E. O'Brien, Maria Gisele Matheus, Kristina Godwin, Amit J. Sood, Anvesh Kompelli, et al. 2019. "Inhibition of MTOR Signaling and Clinical Activity of Rapamycin in Head and Neck Cancer in a Window of Opportunity Trial." *Clinical Cancer Research: An Official Journal of the American Association for Cancer Research* 25 (4): 1156–64. https://doi.org/10.1158/1078-0432.CCR-18-2024.

Deepthi Sogasu, Devaraj Ezhilarasan, and Smiline Girija AS. 2020. "Cancer Stem Cells-Role in Oral Squamous Carcinoma - A Review of Literature." *International Journal of Research in Pharmaceutical Sciences* 11 (SPL3): 153–58. https://doi.org/10.26452/ijrps.v11iSPL3. 2906.

Eppert, Kolja, Katsuto Takenaka, Eric R. Lechman, Levi Waldron, Björn Nilsson, Peter van Galen, Klaus H. Metzeler, et al. 2011. "Stem Cell Gene Expression Programs Influence Clinical Outcome in Human Leukemia." *Nature Medicine* 17 (9): 1086–93. https://doi.org/10.1038/ nm.2415.

Felthaus, O., T. Ettl, M. Gosau, O. Driemel, G. Brockhoff, A. Reck, K. Zeitler, et al. 2011. "Cancer Stem Cell-like Cells from a Single Cell of Oral Squamous Carcinoma Cell Lines." *Biochemical and Biophysical Research Communications* 407 (1): 28–33. https://doi.org/10.1016/j. bbrc.2011.02.084.

Fernando, Romaine I., Mary Litzinger, Paola Trono, Duane H. Hamilton, Jeffrey Schlom, and Claudia Palena. 2010. "The T-Box Transcription Factor Brachyury Promotes Epithelial-Mesenchymal Transition in Human Tumor Cells." *The Journal of Clinical Investigation* 120 (2): 533–44. https://doi.org/10.1172/JCI38379.

Ghuwalewala, Sangeeta, Dishari Ghatak, Pijush Das, Sanjib Dey, Shreya Sarkar, Neyaz Alam, Chinmay K. Panda, and Susanta Roychoudhury. 2016. "CD44(High)CD24(Low) Molecular Signature Determines the Cancer Stem Cell and EMT Phenotype in Oral Squamous Cell Carcinoma." *Stem Cell Research* 16 (2): 405–17. https://doi.org/10.1016/j.scr.2016.02.028.

Gillison, M. L., W. M. Koch, R. B. Capone, M. Spafford, W. H. Westra, L. Wu, M. L. Zahurak, et al. 2000. "Evidence for a Causal Association between Human Papillomavirus and a Subset of Head and Neck Cancers." *Journal of the National Cancer Institute* 92 (9): 709–20. https://doi.org/10.1093/jnci/92.9.709.

Giudice, Fernanda S., Decio S. Pinto, Jacques E. Nör, Cristiane H. Squarize, and Rogerio M. Castilho. 2013. "Inhibition of Histone Deacetylase Impacts Cancer Stem Cells and Induces Epithelial-Mesenchyme Transition of Head and Neck Cancer." *PloS One* 8 (3): e58672. https://doi.org/10.1371/journal.pone.0058672.

Glick, Danielle, Sandra Barth, and Kay F. Macleod. 2010. "Autophagy: Cellular and Molecular Mechanisms." *The Journal of Pathology* 221 (1): 3–12. https://doi.org/10.1002/path.2697.

Grosse-Gehling, Philipp, Christine A. Fargeas, Claudia Dittfeld, Yvette Garbe, Malcolm R. Alison, Denis Corbeil, and Leoni A. Kunz-Schughart. 2013. "CD133 as a Biomarker for Putative Cancer Stem Cells in Solid Tumours: Limitations, Problems and Challenges." *The Journal of Pathology* 229 (3): 355–78. https://doi.org/10.1002/path.4086.

Gu, Feng, Yongjie Ma, Zuping Zhang, Jinghui Zhao, Hisayuki Kobayashi, Lun Zhang, and Li Fu. 2010. "Expression of Stat3 and Notch1 Is Associated with Cisplatin Resistance in Head and Neck Squamous Cell

Carcinoma." *Oncology Reports* 23 (3): 671–76. https://doi.org/10.3892/or_00000683.

Harrison, Hannah, Gillian Farnie, Sacha J. Howell, Rebecca E. Rock, Spyros Stylianou, Keith R. Brennan, Nigel J. Bundred, and Robert B. Clarke. 2010. "Regulation of Breast Cancer Stem Cell Activity by Signaling through the Notch4 Receptor." *Cancer Research* 70 (2): 709–18. https://doi.org/10.1158/0008-5472.CAN-09-1681.

Harsha, Choudhary, Kishore Banik, Hui Li Ang, Sosmitha Girisa, Rajesh Vikkurthi, Dey Parama, Varsha Rana, et al. 2020. "Targeting AKT/MTOR in Oral Cancer: Mechanisms and Advances in Clinical Trials." *International Journal of Molecular Sciences* 21 (9). https://doi.org/10.3390/ijms21093285.

He, Qianting, Zhonghua Liu, Tingting Zhao, Luodan Zhao, Xiaofeng Zhou, and Anxun Wang. 2015. "Bmi1 Drives Stem-Like Properties and Is Associated with Migration, Invasion, and Poor Prognosis in Tongue Squamous Cell Carcinoma." *International Journal of Biological Sciences* 11 (1): 1–10. https://doi.org/10.7150/ijbs.10405.

Hewitt, H. B. 1958. "Studies of the Dissemination and Quantitative Transplantation of a Lymphocytic Leukaemia of CBA Mice." *British Journal of Cancer* 12 (3): 378–401. https://doi.org/10.1038/bjc.1958.47.

Huang, Jhy-Shrian, Chih-Jung Yao, Shuang-En Chuang, Chi-Tai Yeh, Liang-Ming Lee, Ruei-Ming Chen, Wan-Ju Chao, Jacqueline Whang-Peng, and Gi-Ming Lai. 2016. "Honokiol Inhibits Sphere Formation and Xenograft Growth of Oral Cancer Side Population Cells Accompanied with JAK/STAT Signaling Pathway Suppression and Apoptosis Induction." *BMC Cancer* 16 (March). https://doi.org/10. 1186/s12885-016-2265-6.

Icard, Philippe, Laurent Poulain, and Hubert Lincet. 2012. "Understanding the Central Role of Citrate in the Metabolism of Cancer Cells." *Biochimica Et Biophysica Acta* 1825 (1): 111–16. https://doi.org/10.1016/j.bbcan.2011.10.007.

Icard, Philippe, Seth Shulman, Diana Farhat, Jean-Marc Steyaert, Marco Alifano, and Hubert Lincet. 2018. "How the Warburg Effect Supports

Aggressiveness and Drug Resistance of Cancer Cells?" *Drug Resistance Updates: Reviews and Commentaries in Antimicrobial and Anticancer Chemotherapy* 38 (May): 1–11. https://doi.org/10.1016/ j.drup.2018.03.001.

Ingham, P. W., and A. P. McMahon. 2001. "Hedgehog Signaling in Animal Development: Paradigms and Principles." *Genes & Development* 15 (23): 3059–87. https://doi.org/10.1101/gad.938601.

Kalluri, Raghu, and Robert A. Weinberg. 2009. "The Basics of Epithelial-Mesenchymal Transition." *The Journal of Clinical Investigation* 119 (6): 1420–28. https://doi.org/10.1172/JCI39104.

Kolenda, Tomasz, Kacper Guglas, Marcel Ryś, Marta Bogaczyńska, Anna Teresiak, Renata Bliźniak, Izabela Łasińska, Jacek Mackiewicz, and Katarzyna M. Lamperska. 2017. "Biological Role of Long Non-Coding RNA in Head and Neck Cancers." *Reports of Practical Oncology and Radiotherapy: Journal of Greatpoland Cancer Center in Poznan and Polish Society of Radiation Oncology* 22 (5): 378–88. https://doi.org/10.1016/j.rpor.2017.07.001.

Kong, Ying, Yuanqiu Peng, Yuan Liu, Hong Xin, Xia Zhan, and Wenfu Tan. 2015. "Twist1 and Snail Link Hedgehog Signaling to Tumor-Initiating Cell-like Properties and Acquired Chemoresistance Independently of ABC Transporters." *Stem Cells (Dayton, Ohio)* 33 (4): 1063–74. https://doi.org/10.1002/stem.1955.

Krishnamurthy, S., and J. E. Nör. 2012. "Head and Neck Cancer Stem Cells." *Journal of Dental Research* 91 (4): 334–40. https://doi.org/10.1177/0022034511423393.

Krishnamurthy, Sudha, and Jacques E. Nör. 2013. "Orosphere Assay: A Method for Propagation of Head and Neck Cancer Stem Cells." *Head & Neck* 35 (7): 1015–21. https://doi.org/10.1002/hed.23076.

Kuo, Selena Z., Katherine J. Blair, Elham Rahimy, Alan Kiang, Eric Abhold, Jian-Bing Fan, Jessica Wang-Rodriguez, Xabier Altuna, and Weg M. Ongkeko. 2012. "Salinomycin Induces Cell Death and Differentiation in Head and Neck Squamous Cell Carcinoma Stem Cells despite Activation of Epithelial-Mesenchymal Transition and Akt." *BMC*

Cancer 12 (November): 556. https://doi.org/10.1186/1471-2407-12-556.

Kuroda, Hiromasa, Naito Kurio, Tsuyoshi Shimo, Kenichi Matsumoto, Masanori Masui, Kiyofumi Takabatake, Tatsuo Okui, et al. 2017. "Oral Squamous Cell Carcinoma-Derived Sonic Hedgehog Promotes Angiogenesis." *Anticancer Research* 37 (12): 6731–37. https://doi.org/10.21873/anticanres.12132.

Lai, Stephen Y., and Faye M. Johnson. 2010. "Defining the Role of the JAK-STAT Pathway in Head and Neck and Thoracic Malignancies: Implications for Future Therapeutic Approaches." *Drug Resistance Updates: Reviews and Commentaries in Antimicrobial and Anticancer Chemotherapy* 13 (3): 67–78. https://doi.org/10.1016/j.drup.2010.04.001.

Le, Phuong N., Stephen B. Keysar, Bettina Miller, Justin R. Eagles, Tugs-Saikhan Chimed, Julie Reisinger, Karina E. Gomez, et al. 2019. "Wnt Signaling Dynamics in Head and Neck Squamous Cell Cancer Tumor-Stroma Interactions." *Molecular Carcinogenesis* 58 (3): 398–410. https://doi.org/10.1002/mc.22937.

Lee, Sang H., Sung I. Do, Hyun J. Lee, Hyun J. Kang, Bon S. Koo, and Young C. Lim. 2016. "Notch1 Signaling Contributes to Stemness in Head and Neck Squamous Cell Carcinoma." *Laboratory Investigation; a Journal of Technical Methods and Pathology* 96 (5): 508–16. https://doi.org/10.1038/labinvest.2015.163.

Lee, Sung Hee, Hannah S. Hong, Zi Xiao Liu, Reuben H. Kim, Mo K. Kang, No-Hee Park, and Ki-Hyuk Shin. 2012. "TNFα Enhances Cancer Stem Cell-like Phenotype via Notch-Hes1 Activation in Oral Squamous Cell Carcinoma Cells." *Biochemical and Biophysical Research Communications* 424 (1): 58–64. https://doi.org/10.1016/j. bbrc.2012.06.065.

Lee, Sung Hee, Nicole Rigas, Charlotte Ellen Martin, Anthony Nguyen, Mo K. Kang, No-Hee Park, Reuben H. Kim, and Ki-Hyuk Shin. 2021. "Zoledronic Acid Impairs Oral Cancer Stem Cells by Reducing CCL3." *Oncology Reports* 45 (1): 291–98. https://doi.org/10.3892/or.2020.7835.

Li, Da-Wei, Pin Dong, Fei Wang, Xin-Wei Chen, Cheng-Zhi Xu, and Liang Zhou. 2013. "Hypoxia Induced Multidrug Resistance of Laryngeal Cancer Cells via Hypoxia-Inducible Factor-1α." *Asian Pacific Journal of Cancer Prevention: APJCP* 14 (8): 4853–58. https://doi.org/10.7314/apjcp.2013.14.8.4853.

Li, Youzhi, Harry A. Rogoff, Sarah Keates, Yuan Gao, Sylaja Murikipudi, Keith Mikule, David Leggett, Wei Li, Arthur B. Pardee, and Chiang J. Li. 2015. "Suppression of Cancer Relapse and Metastasis by Inhibiting Cancer Stemness." *Proceedings of the National Academy of Sciences of the United States of America* 112 (6): 1839–44. https://doi.org/10.1073/pnas.1424171112.

Lin, Feng, Li Gao, Zhenyu Su, Xiaofang Cao, Yuanbo Zhan, Ying Li, and Bin Zhang. 2018. "Knockdown of KPNA2 Inhibits Autophagy in Oral Squamous Cell Carcinoma Cell Lines by Blocking P53 Nuclear Translocation." *Oncology Reports* 40 (1): 179–94. https://doi.org/10.3892/or.2018.6451.

Lin, Qun, and Zhong Yun. 2010. "Impact of the Hypoxic Tumor Microenvironment on the Regulation of Cancer Stem Cell Characteristics." *Cancer Biology & Therapy* 9 (12): 949–56. https://doi.org/10.4161/cbt.9.12.12347.

Liu, Xue, Yu Fu, Jiadong Huang, Meng Wu, Zhenxing Zhang, Rongyao Xu, Ping Zhang, Shouwei Zhao, Laikui Liu, and Hongbing Jiang. 2019. "ADAR1 Promotes the Epithelial-to-Mesenchymal Transition and Stem-like Cell Phenotype of Oral Cancer by Facilitating Oncogenic MicroRNA Maturation." *Journal of Experimental & Clinical Cancer Research: CR* 38 (1): 315. https://doi.org/10.1186/ s13046-019-1300-2.

Lv, Xiao-Xi, Xiao-Yu Zheng, Jiao-Jiao Yu, Hua-Rui Ma, Cheng Hua, and Run-Tao Gao. 2020. "EGFR Enhances the Stemness and Progression of Oral Cancer through Inhibiting Autophagic Degradation of SOX2." *Cancer Medicine* 9 (3): 1131–40. https://doi.org/10.1002/cam4.2772.

Lv, Zhiyong, Ye Yang, and Chunyan Yang. 2020. "Integrin A7 Correlates with Worse Clinical Features and Prognosis, and Its Knockdown Inhibits Cell Proliferation and Stemness in Tongue Squamous Cell

Carcinoma." *International Journal of Oncology* 56 (1): 69–84. https://doi.org/10.3892/ijo.2019.4927.

M, Pentenero, Gandolfo S, and Carrozzo M. 2005. "Importance of Tumor Thickness and Depth of Invasion in Nodal Involvement and Prognosis of Oral Squamous Cell Carcinoma: A Review of the Literature." *Head & Neck* 27 (12). https://doi.org/10.1002/hed.20275.

Major, Aidan G., Luke P. Pitty, and Camile S. Farah. 2013. "Cancer Stem Cell Markers in Head and Neck Squamous Cell Carcinoma." *Stem Cells International* 2013: 319489. https://doi.org/10.1155/2013/ 319489.

Masui, Takashi, Ichiro Ota, Jong-In Yook, Shinji Mikami, Katsunari Yane, Toshiaki Yamanaka, and Hiroshi Hosoi. 2014. "Snail-Induced Epithelial-Mesenchymal Transition Promotes Cancer Stem Cell-like Phenotype in Head and Neck Cancer Cells." *International Journal of Oncology* 44 (3): 693–99. https://doi.org/10.3892/ijo.2013.2225.

Mehrotra, R., and S. Yadav. 2006. "Oral Squamous Cell Carcinoma: Etiology, Pathogenesis and Prognostic Value of Genomic Alterations." *Indian Journal of Cancer* 43 (2): 60–66. https://doi.org/10.4103/0019-509x.25886.

Melo, Felipe De Sousa E, Louis Vermeulen, Evelyn Fessler, and Jan Paul Medema. 2013. "Cancer Heterogeneity—a Multifaceted View." *EMBO Reports* 14 (8): 686–95. https://doi.org/10.1038/embor.2013.92.

Meurette, Olivier, and Patrick Mehlen. 2018. "Notch Signaling in the Tumor Microenvironment." *Cancer Cell* 34 (4): 536–48. https://doi.org/10.1016/j.ccell.2018.07.009.

Michifuri, Yoshitaka, Yoshihiko Hirohashi, Toshihiko Torigoe, Akihiro Miyazaki, Junichi Kobayashi, Takanori Sasaki, Jyunki Fujino, et al. 2012. "High Expression of ALDH1 and SOX2 Diffuse Staining Pattern of Oral Squamous Cell Carcinomas Correlates to Lymph Node Metastasis." *Pathology International* 62 (10): 684–89. https://doi.org/10.1111/j.1440-1827.2012.02851.x.

Min, Anjie, Chao Zhu, Jingyi Wang, Shuping Peng, Cijun Shuai, Shan Gao, Zhangui Tang, and Tong Su. 2015. "Focal Adhesion Kinase Knockdown in Carcinoma-Associated Fibroblasts Inhibits Oral Squamous Cell Carcinoma Metastasis via Downregulating MCP-1/CCL2 Expression."

Journal of Biochemical and Molecular Toxicology 29 (2): 70–76. https://doi.org/10.1002/jbt.21669.

Mirhashemi, Majid, Narges Ghazi, Nasrollah Saghravanian, Ali Taghipour, and Farnaz Mohajertehran. 2020. "Evaluation of CD24 and CD44 as Cancer Stem Cell Markers in Squamous Cell Carcinoma and Epithelial Dysplasia of the Oral Cavity by Q- RT-PCR." *Dental Research Journal* 17 (3): 208–12.

Naik, Prajna Paramita, Durgesh Nandini Das, Prashanta Kumar Panda, Subhadip Mukhopadhyay, Niharika Sinha, Prakash Priyadarshi Praharaj, Rajesh Agarwal, and Sujit Kumar Bhutia. 2016. "Implications of Cancer Stem Cells in Developing Therapeutic Resistance in Oral Cancer." *Oral Oncology* 62 (November): 122–35. https://doi.org/10.1016/j.oraloncology.2016.10.008.

Nair, Sindhu, Hoa Q. Trummell, Rajani Rajbhandari, Nanda K. Thudi, Susan E. Nozell, Jason M. Warram, Christopher D. Willey, et al. 2020. "Novel EGFR Ectodomain Mutations Associated with Ligand-Independent Activation and Cetuximab Resistance in Head and Neck Cancer." *PloS One* 15 (2): e0229077. https://doi.org/10.1371/journal. pone.0229077.

Nguyen, Long V., Robert Vanner, Peter Dirks, and Connie J. Eaves. 2012. "Cancer Stem Cells: An Evolving Concept." *Nature Reviews. Cancer* 12 (2): 133–43. https://doi.org/10.1038/nrc3184.

Niehrs, Christof. 2012. "The Complex World of WNT Receptor Signalling." *Nature Reviews. Molecular Cell Biology* 13 (12): 767–79. https://doi.org/10.1038/nrm3470.

Nusse, Roel, and Hans Clevers. 2017. "Wnt/β-Catenin Signaling, Disease, and Emerging Therapeutic Modalities." *Cell* 169 (6): 985–99. https://doi.org/10.1016/j.cell.2017.05.016.

O'Brien, Catherine Adell, Antonija Kreso, and Catriona H. M. Jamieson. 2010. "Cancer Stem Cells and Self-Renewal." *Clinical Cancer Research: An Official Journal of the American Association for Cancer Research* 16 (12): 3113–20. https://doi.org/10.1158/1078-0432.CCR-09-2824.

Ota, Ichiro, Takashi Masui, Miyako Kurihara, Jong-In Yook, Shinji Mikami, Takahiro Kimura, Keiji Shimada, et al. 2016. "Snail-Induced EMT

Promotes Cancer Stem Cell-like Properties in Head and Neck Cancer Cells." *Oncology Reports* 35 (1): 261–66. https://doi.org/10.3892/or.2015.4348.

Pai, Shin, Oluwaseun Adebayo Bamodu, Yen-Kuang Lin, Chun-Shu Lin, Pei-Yi Chu, Ming-Hsien Chien, Liang-Shun Wang, Michael Hsiao, Chi-Tai Yeh, and Jo-Ting Tsai. 2019. "CD47-SIRPα Signaling Induces Epithelial-Mesenchymal Transition and Cancer Stemness and Links to a Poor Prognosis in Patients with Oral Squamous Cell Carcinoma." *Cells* 8 (12). https://doi.org/10.3390/cells8121658.

Pannuti, Antonio, Kimberly Foreman, Paola Rizzo, Clodia Osipo, Todd Golde, Barbara Osborne, and Lucio Miele. 2010. "Targeting Notch to Target Cancer Stem Cells." *Clinical Cancer Research: An Official Journal of the American Association for Cancer Research* 16 (12): 3141–52. https://doi.org/10.1158/1078-0432.CCR-09-2823.

Pardal, Ricardo, Michael F. Clarke, and Sean J. Morrison. 2003. "Applying the Principles of Stem-Cell Biology to Cancer." *Nature Reviews. Cancer* 3 (12): 895–902. https://doi.org/10.1038/nrc1232.

Patni, Anjali P., M. K. Harishankar, Joel P. Joseph, Bhuvanadas Sreeshma, Rama Jayaraj, and Arikketh Devi. 2021. "Comprehending the Crosstalk between Notch, Wnt and Hedgehog Signaling Pathways in Oral Squamous Cell Carcinoma - Clinical Implications." *Cellular Oncology (Dordrecht)*, March. https://doi.org/10.1007/s13402-021-00591-3.

Peña-Oyarzún, Daniel, Montserrat Reyes, María Paz Hernández-Cáceres, Catalina Kretschmar, Eugenia Morselli, Cesar A. Ramirez-Sarmiento, Sergio Lavandero, Vicente A. Torres, and Alfredo Criollo. 2020. "Role of Autophagy in the Microenvironment of Oral Squamous Cell Carcinoma." *Frontiers in Oncology* 10 (December). https://doi.org/10.3389/fonc.2020.602661.

Peng, Fusen, Hailin Zhang, Youhong Du, and Pingqing Tan. 2015. "MiR-23a Promotes Cisplatin Chemoresistance and Protects against Cisplatin-Induced Apoptosis in Tongue Squamous Cell Carcinoma Cells through Twist." *Oncology Reports* 33 (2): 942–50. https://doi.org/10.3892/or.2014.3664.

Perez, Aymee, David M. Neskey, Judy Wen, Lutecia Pereira, Erika P. Reategui, W. Jarrard Goodwin, Kermit L. Carraway, and Elizabeth J. Franzmann. 2013. "CD44 Interacts with EGFR and Promotes Head and Neck Squamous Cell Carcinoma Initiation and Progression." *Oral Oncology* 49 (4): 306–13. https://doi.org/10.1016/j.oraloncology.2012.11.009.

Prince, M. E., R. Sivanandan, A. Kaczorowski, G. T. Wolf, M. J. Kaplan, P. Dalerba, I. L. Weissman, M. F. Clarke, and L. E. Ailles. 2007. "Identification of a Subpopulation of Cells with Cancer Stem Cell Properties in Head and Neck Squamous Cell Carcinoma." *Proceedings of the National Academy of Sciences of the United States of America* 104 (3): 973–78. https://doi.org/10.1073/pnas.0610117104.

Pukkila, M. J., J. A. Virtaniemi, E. J. Kumpulainen, R. T. Pirinen, R. T. Johansson, H. J. Valtonen, M. T. Juhola, and V. M. Kosma. 2001. "Nuclear Beta Catenin Expression Is Related to Unfavourable Outcome in Oropharyngeal and Hypopharyngeal Squamous Cell Carcinoma." *Journal of Clinical Pathology* 54 (1): 42–47. https://doi.org/10.1136/jcp.54.1.42.

Rebay, I., R. J. Fleming, R. G. Fehon, L. Cherbas, P. Cherbas, and S. Artavanis-Tsakonas. 1991. "Specific EGF Repeats of Notch Mediate Interactions with Delta and Serrate: Implications for Notch as a Multifunctional Receptor." *Cell* 67 (4): 687–99. https://doi.org/10.1016/0092-8674(91)90064-6.

Reya, T., S. J. Morrison, M. F. Clarke, and I. L. Weissman. 2001. "Stem Cells, Cancer, and Cancer Stem Cells." *Nature* 414 (6859): 105–11. https://doi.org/10.1038/35102167.

Reyes, Montserrat, Tania Flores, Diego Betancur, Daniel Peña-Oyarzún, and Vicente A. Torres. 2020. "Wnt/β-Catenin Signaling in Oral Carcinogenesis." *International Journal of Molecular Sciences* 21 (13). https://doi.org/10.3390/ijms21134682.

Roche, Joëlle. 2018. "The Epithelial-to-Mesenchymal Transition in Cancer." *Cancers* 10 (2). https://doi.org/10.3390/cancers10020052.

Roy, Souvick, Madhabananda Kar, Shomereeta Roy, Swatishree Padhi, Arka Saha, and Birendranath Banerjee. 2019. "KLF4 Expression in the

Surgical Cut Margin Is Associated with Disease Relapse of Oral Squamous Cell Carcinoma." *Oral Surgery, Oral Medicine, Oral Pathology and Oral Radiology* 128 (2): 154–65. https://doi.org/10.1016/j.oooo.2019.02.021.

Ryott, Michael, Darawalee Wangsa, Kerstin Heselmeyer-Haddad, Johan Lindholm, Göran Elmberger, Gert Auer, Elisabeth Avall Lundqvist, Thomas Ried, and Eva Munck-Wikland. 2009. "EGFR Protein Overexpression and Gene Copy Number Increases in Oral Tongue Squamous Cell Carcinoma." *European Journal of Cancer (Oxford, England: 1990)* 45 (9): 1700–1708. https://doi.org/10.1016/j.ejca.2009.02.027.

Sakakura, Koichi, Hideyuki Takahashi, Kyoichi Kaira, Minoru Toyoda, Tetsunari Oyama, and Kazuaki Chikamatsu. 2015. "Immunological Significance of the Accumulation of Autophagy Components in Oral Squamous Cell Carcinoma." *Cancer Science* 106 (1): 1–8. https://doi.org/10.1111/cas.12559.

Scheel, Christina, and Robert A. Weinberg. 2012. "Cancer Stem Cells and Epithelial-Mesenchymal Transition: Concepts and Molecular Links." *Seminars in Cancer Biology* 22 (5–6): 396–403. https://doi.org/10.1016/j.semcancer.2012.04.001.

Schulz, Dominik, Markus Wirth, Guido Piontek, Anna Maria Stefanie Buchberger, Jürgen Schlegel, Rudolf Reiter, Gabriele Multhoff, and Anja Pickhard. 2016. "HNSCC Cells Resistant to EGFR Pathway Inhibitors Are Hypermutated and Sensitive to DNA Damaging Substances." *American Journal of Cancer Research* 6 (9): 1963–75.

Sen, Malabika, Sonali Joyce, Mary Panahandeh, Changyou Li, Sufi M. Thomas, Jessica Maxwell, Lin Wang, William E. Gooding, Daniel E. Johnson, and Jennifer R. Grandis. 2012. "Targeting Stat3 Abrogates EGFR Inhibitor Resistance in Cancer." *Clinical Cancer Research: An Official Journal of the American Association for Cancer Research* 18 (18): 4986–96. https://doi.org/10.1158/1078-0432.CCR-12-0792.

Shackleton, Mark, Elsa Quintana, Eric R. Fearon, and Sean J. Morrison. 2009. "Heterogeneity in Cancer: Cancer Stem Cells versus Clonal

Evolution." *Cell* 138 (5): 822–29. https://doi.org/10.1016/j.cell. 2009.08.017.

Shimoda, Masayuki, Masahide Ota, and Yasunori Okada. 2018. "Isolation of Cancer Stem Cells by Side Population Method." *Methods in Molecular Biology (Clifton, N.J.)* 1692: 49–59. https://doi.org/10.1007/978-1-4939-7401-6_5.

Silva, Sabrina Daniela da, Moulay A. Alaoui-Jamali, Fernando Augusto Soares, Dirce Maria Carraro, Helena Paula Brentani, Michael Hier, Silvia Regina Rogatto, and Luiz Paulo Kowalski. 2014. "TWIST1 Is a Molecular Marker for a Poor Prognosis in Oral Cancer and Represents a Potential Therapeutic Target." *Cancer* 120 (3): 352–62. https://doi.org/10.1002/cncr.28404.

Silva, Sabrina Daniela da, Michael Hier, Alex Mlynarek, Luiz Paulo Kowalski, and Moulay A. Alaoui-Jamali. 2012. "Recurrent Oral Cancer: Current and Emerging Therapeutic Approaches." *Frontiers in Pharmacology* 3: 149. https://doi.org/10.3389/fphar.2012.00149.

Skrzypek, Klaudia, and Marcin Majka. 2020. "Interplay among SNAIL Transcription Factor, MicroRNAs, Long Non-Coding RNAs, and Circular RNAs in the Regulation of Tumor Growth and Metastasis." *Cancers* 12 (1). https://doi.org/10.3390/cancers12010209.

Stern, Robert, Svetlana Shuster, Birgit A. Neudecker, and Bent Formby. 2002. "Lactate Stimulates Fibroblast Expression of Hyaluronan and CD44: The Warburg Effect Revisited." *Experimental Cell Research* 276 (1): 24–31. https://doi.org/10.1006/excr.2002.5508.

Stolpe, Anja van de. 2013. "On the Origin and Destination of Cancer Stem Cells: A Conceptual Evaluation." *American Journal of Cancer Research* 3 (1): 107–16.

Takahashi-Yanaga, Fumi, and Michael Kahn. 2010. "Targeting Wnt Signaling: Can We Safely Eradicate Cancer Stem Cells?" *Clinical Cancer Research: An Official Journal of the American Association for Cancer Research* 16 (12): 3153–62. https://doi.org/10.1158/1078-0432.CCR-09-2943.

Takezaki, Tatsuya, Takuichiro Hide, Hiromi Takanaga, Hideo Nakamura, Jun-Ichi Kuratsu, and Toru Kondo. 2011. "Essential Role of the

Hedgehog Signaling Pathway in Human Glioma-Initiating Cells." *Cancer Science* 102 (7): 1306–12. https://doi.org/10.1111/j.1349-7006.2011.01943.x.

Talukdar, Sarmistha, Luni Emdad, Swadesh K. Das, and Paul B. Fisher. 2020. "EGFR: An Essential Receptor Tyrosine Kinase-Regulator of Cancer Stem Cells." *Advances in Cancer Research* 147: 161–88. https://doi.org/10.1016/bs.acr.2020.04.003.

Tanaka, N, T Odajima, K Ogi, T Ikeda, and M Satoh. 2003. "Expression of E-Cadherin, α-Catenin, and β-Catenin in the Process of Lymph Node Metastasis in Oral Squamous Cell Carcinoma." *British Journal of Cancer* 89 (3): 557–63. https://doi.org/10.1038/sj.bjc.6601124.

Tang, Carol, Beng T. Ang, and Shazib Pervaiz. 2007. "Cancer Stem Cell: Target for Anti-Cancer Therapy." *FASEB Journal: Official Publication of the Federation of American Societies for Experimental Biology* 21 (14): 3777–85. https://doi.org/10.1096/fj.07-8560rev.

Thierauf, Julia, Johannes Adrian Veit, and Jochen Hess. 2017. "Epithelial-to-Mesenchymal Transition in the Pathogenesis and Therapy of Head and Neck Cancer." *Cancers* 9 (7). https://doi.org/10.3390/cancers 9070076.

Tong, Wei-Wei, Guang-Hui Tong, and Yong Liu. 2018. "Cancer Stem Cells and Hypoxia-Inducible Factors (Review)." *International Journal of Oncology* 53 (2): 469–76. https://doi.org/10.3892/ijo.2018.4417.

Vander Broek, R., S. Mohan, D. F. Eytan, Z. Chen, and C. Van Waes. 2015. "The PI3K/Akt/MTOR Axis in Head and Neck Cancer: Functions, Aberrations, Cross-Talk, and Therapies." *Oral Diseases* 21 (7): 815–25. https://doi.org/10.1111/odi.12206.

Vander Heiden, Matthew G., Lewis C. Cantley, and Craig B. Thompson. 2009. "Understanding the Warburg Effect: The Metabolic Requirements of Cell Proliferation." *Science (New York, N.Y.)* 324 (5930): 1029–33. https://doi.org/10.1126/science.1160809.

Varjosalo, Markku, and Jussi Taipale. 2007. "Hedgehog Signaling." *Journal of Cell Science* 120 (Pt 1): 3–6. https://doi.org/10.1242/jcs. 03309.

Varun, BR, P Jayanthi, and Pratibha Ramani. 2020. "Cancer Stem Cells: A Comprehensive Review on Identification and Therapeutic

Implications." *Journal of Oral and Maxillofacial Pathology : JOMFP* 24 (1): 190. https://doi.org/10.4103/jomfp.JOMFP_336_19.

Vermeulen, Louis, Felipe De Sousa E Melo, Maartje van der Heijden, Kate Cameron, Joan H. de Jong, Tijana Borovski, Jurriaan B. Tuynman, et al. 2010. "Wnt Activity Defines Colon Cancer Stem Cells and Is Regulated by the Microenvironment." *Nature Cell Biology* 12 (5): 468–76. https://doi.org/10.1038/ncb2048.

Wang, Jianbo, Tanvi Sinha, and Anthony Wynshaw-Boris. 2012. "Wnt Signaling in Mammalian Development: Lessons from Mouse Genetics." *Cold Spring Harbor Perspectives in Biology* 4 (5). https://doi.org/10.1101/cshperspect.a007963.

Wang, Steven J., and Lilly Y. W. Bourguignon. 2006. "Hyaluronan and the Interaction between CD44 and Epidermal Growth Factor Receptor in Oncogenic Signaling and Chemotherapy Resistance in Head and Neck Cancer." *Archives of Otolaryngology--Head & Neck Surgery* 132 (7): 771–78. https://doi.org/10.1001/archotol.132.7.771.

Warburg, O. 1956. "On the Origin of Cancer Cells." *Science (New York, N.Y.)* 123 (3191): 309–14. https://doi.org/10.1126/science.123.3191.309.

Warrier, S., G. Bhuvanalakshmi, F. Arfuso, G. Rajan, M. Millward, and A. Dharmarajan. 2014. "Cancer Stem-like Cells from Head and Neck Cancers Are Chemosensitized by the Wnt Antagonist, SFRP4, by Inducing Apoptosis, Decreasing Stemness, Drug Resistance and Epithelial to Mesenchymal Transition." *Cancer Gene Therapy* 21 (9): 381–88. https://doi.org/10.1038/cgt.2014.42.

Warrier, Sudha, Senthil Kumar Balu, Alan Prem Kumar, Michael Millward, and Arunasalam Dharmarajan. 2013. "Wnt Antagonist, Secreted Frizzled-Related Protein 4 (SFRP4), Increases Chemotherapeutic Response of Glioma Stem-like Cells." *Oncology Research* 21 (2): 93–102. https://doi.org/10.3727/096504013X13786 659070154.

Willey, Christopher D., Joshua C. Anderson, Hoa Q. Trummell, Faris Naji, Rik de Wijn, Eddy S. Yang, Markus Bredel, Nanda K. Thudi, and James A. Bonner. 2019. "Differential Escape Mechanisms in Cetuximab-Resistant Head and Neck Cancer Cells." *Biochemical and Biophysical*

Research Communications 517 (1): 36–42. https://doi.org/10.1016/j.bbrc.2019.06.159.

Wu, Ming-Heng, Hsiao-Chin Hong, Tse-Ming Hong, Wei-Fan Chiang, Ying-Tai Jin, and Yuh-Ling Chen. 2011. "Targeting Galectin-1 in Carcinoma-Associated Fibroblasts Inhibits Oral Squamous Cell Carcinoma Metastasis by Downregulating MCP-1/CCL2 Expression." *Clinical Cancer Research: An Official Journal of the American Association for Cancer Research* 17 (6): 1306–16. https://doi.org/10.1158/1078-0432.CCR-10-1824.

Xu, Qijin, Xiangpeng Yuan, Gentao Liu, Keith L. Black, and John S. Yu. 2008. "Hedgehog Signaling Regulates Brain Tumor-Initiating Cell Proliferation and Portends Shorter Survival for Patients with PTEN-Coexpressing Glioblastomas." *Stem Cells (Dayton, Ohio)* 26 (12): 3018–26. https://doi.org/10.1634/stemcells.2008-0459.

Xu, Qilin, Qunzhou Zhang, Yasutaka Ishida, Souren Hajjar, Xudong Tang, Haoran Shi, Chi V. Dang, and Anh D. Le. 2017. "EGF Induces Epithelial-Mesenchymal Transition and Cancer Stem-like Cell Properties in Human Oral Cancer Cells via Promoting Warburg Effect." *Oncotarget* 8 (6): 9557–71. https://doi.org/10.18632/ oncotarget.13771.

Yan, Huiwen, and Pengcheng Bu. 2018. "Non-Coding RNAs in Cancer Stem Cells." *Cancer Letters* 421 (May): 121–26. https://doi.org/10.1016/j.canlet.2018.01.027.

Yang, Muh-Hwa, Dennis Shin-Shian Hsu, Hsei-Wei Wang, Hsiao-Jung Wang, Hsin-Yi Lan, Wen-Hao Yang, Chi-Hung Huang, et al. 2010. "Bmi1 Is Essential in Twist1-Induced Epithelial-Mesenchymal Transition." *Nature Cell Biology* 12 (10): 982–92. https://doi.org/10.1038/ncb2099.

Yao, Chih-Jung, Gi-Ming Lai, Chi-Tai Yeh, Ming-Tang Lai, Ping-Hsiao Shih, Wan-Ju Chao, Jacqueline Whang-Peng, Shuang-En Chuang, and Tung-Yuan Lai. 2013. "Honokiol Eliminates Human Oral Cancer Stem-Like Cells Accompanied with Suppression of Wnt/ β -Catenin Signaling and Apoptosis Induction." *Evidence-Based Complementary and Alternative Medicine: ECAM* 2013: 146136. https://doi.org/10.1155/2013/146136.

Yj, Chen, Lin Sc, Kao T, Chang Cs, Hong Ps, Shieh Tm, and Chang Kw. 2004. "Genome-Wide Profiling of Oral Squamous Cell Carcinoma." *The Journal of Pathology* 204 (3). https://doi.org/10.1002/path.1640.

Yokogi, Satoshi, Toshiaki Tsubota, Keita Kanki, Junya Azumi, Noriko Itaba, Hiroyuki Oka, Minoru Morimoto, Kazuo Ryoke, and Goshi Shiota. 2016. "Wnt/Beta-Catenin Signal Inhibitor HC-1 Sensitizes Oral Squamous Cell Carcinoma Cells to 5-Fluorouracil through Reduction of CD44-Positive Population." *Yonago Acta Medica* 59 (2): 93–99.

Yoon, Hye-Jung, Ji-Soo Hong, Wui-Jung Shin, Yoo-Jin Lee, Kyoung-Ok Hong, Jae-Il Lee, Sam-Pyo Hong, and Seong-Doo Hong. 2011. "The Role of Cripto-1 in the Tumorigenesis and Progression of Oral Squamous Cell Carcinoma." *Oral Oncology* 47 (11): 1023–31. https://doi.org/10.1016/j.oraloncology.2011.07.019.

Yoshihama, Rumi, Koujiro Yamaguchi, Ikumi Imajyo, Mariko Mine, Naomi Hiyake, Naonari Akimoto, Yosuke Kobayashi, et al. 2016. "Expression Levels of SOX2, KLF4 and Brachyury Transcription Factors Are Associated with Metastasis and Poor Prognosis in Oral Squamous Cell Carcinoma." *Oncology Letters* 11 (2): 1435–46. https://doi.org/10.3892/ol.2015.4047.

Yu, Cheng-Chia, Fang-Wei Hu, Chuan-Hang Yu, and Ming-Yung Chou. 2016. "Targeting CD133 in the Enhancement of Chemosensitivity in Oral Squamous Cell Carcinoma-Derived Side Population Cancer Stem Cells." *Head & Neck* 38 Suppl 1 (April): E231-238. https://doi.org/10.1002/hed.23975.

Yu, Ziwei, Paul M. Weinberger, Elayne Provost, Bruce G. Haffty, Clarence Sasaki, J. Joe, R. L. Camp, D. L. Rimm, and Amanda Psyrri. 2005. "Beta-Catenin Functions Mainly as an Adhesion Molecule in Patients with Squamous Cell Cancer of the Head and Neck." *Clinical Cancer Research: An Official Journal of the American Association for Cancer Research* 11 (7): 2471–77. https://doi.org/10.1158/1078-0432.CCR-04-2199.

Zhang, Qunzhou, Shihong Shi, Yun Yen, Jimmy Brown, Joseph Quoc Ta, and Anh D. Le. 2010. "A Subpopulation of CD133(+) Cancer Stem-like Cells Characterized in Human Oral Squamous Cell Carcinoma Confer

Resistance to Chemotherapy." *Cancer Letters* 289 (2): 151–60. https://doi.org/10.1016/j.canlet.2009.08.010.

Zhang, Zhaocheng, Zhihong Dong, Isabel S. Lauxen, Manoel Sant'Ana Filho, and Jacques E. Nör. 2014. "Endothelial Cell-Secreted EGF Induces Epithelial to Mesenchymal Transition and Endows Head and Neck Cancer Cells with Stem-like Phenotype." *Cancer Research* 74 (10): 2869–81. https://doi.org/10.1158/0008-5472.CAN-13-2032.

Zhao, Zhi-Li, Lu Zhang, Cong-Fa Huang, Si-Rui Ma, Lin-Lin Bu, Jian-Feng Liu, Guang-Tao Yu, et al. 2016. "NOTCH1 Inhibition Enhances the Efficacy of Conventional Chemotherapeutic Agents by Targeting Head Neck Cancer Stem Cell." *Scientific Reports* 6 (April): 24704. https://doi.org/10.1038/srep24704.

Zheng, Yang, Chundi Wang, An Song, Feng Jiang, Junbo Zhou, Gang Li, Wei Zhang, et al. 2020. "CMTM6 Promotes Cell Proliferation and Invasion in Oral Squamous Cell Carcinoma by Interacting with NRP1." *American Journal of Cancer Research* 10 (6): 1691–1709.

Zhu, Qing-Qing, Chenhui Ma, Qian Wang, Yong Song, and Tangfeng Lv. 2016. "The Role of TWIST1 in Epithelial-Mesenchymal Transition and Cancers." *Tumour Biology: The Journal of the International Society for Oncodevelopmental Biology and Medicine* 37 (1): 185–97. https://doi.org/10.1007/s13277-015-4450-7.

In: Oral Squamous Cell Carcinoma
Editor: Matthew Rabin

ISBN: 978-1-53619-895-9

Chapter 4

DIAGNOSTICS AND THERAPEUTIC APPLICATIONS OF NANOTECHNOLOGY AND NANOMEDICINE IN ORAL SQUAMOUS CELL CARCINOMA

Rajib Dhar, Gauresh Gurudas Shivji and Arikketh Devi**, PhD

Cancer Biology and Stem Cell Biology Lab,
Department of Genetic Engineering,
SRM Institute of Science and Technology, Tamil Nadu, India

ABSTRACT

Oral squamous cell carcinoma (OSCC) is the most common cancer worldwide. Several factors influence OSCC, tobacco use having a high impact on OSCC development. The prevention of OSCC may be possible by reducing exposure to the risk factors of OSCC. OSCC is the sixth most deadly cancer globally, owing to the drawback of the traditional approach in OSCC treatment and failure of diagnosis at an early stage. The primary

* Corresponding Author's E-mail: devia@srmist.edu.in.

stage of detection and a sedentary lifestyle mainly contributes to the morbidity and mortality of OSCC patients. In this scenario, nanotechnology gives a new direction for the treatment and diagnosis of oral cancer. Nanomedicine shows a highly promising result with low toxicity. The toxicity of nanomaterial can be controlled by improving functionalization and systematically minimizing toxicity. As a result, nanomaterial and nanomedicine becomes more biologically compatible. Nanomedicine-based targeted drug delivery to the tumor site releases therapeutic agents most effectively, possibly increasing the efficacy of nanomedicine. This book chapter aims to cover the recent developments in Nanotechnology-based drug delivery systems, advance nanomedicines (Nano-capsules, Gold nanoparticles, Quantum dots, and Carbon nanotubes) and their diagnostics as well as therapeutic applications in OSCC.

Keyword: oral squamous cell carcinoma, nanomedicine, drug delivery

INTRODUCTION

Cancer is a disease of gene alterations attributed to specific mutations that results in an abnormal increase in the number of cells, leading to many complications resulting in a malignant tumor or neoplasm. Cancer is one of the most complex and heterogeneous disease that has continued to affect the human population for many decades (Stratton et al., 2014). There were about 14 million cases and 8 million deaths in 2012, and in the year 2020, it peaked up to 19.3 million cases and 10 million cancer deaths (Stewart et al., 2014) (Sung et al., 2020). Cancer treatment strategies mostly include cytotoxic chemotherapy, radiation therapy and surgical removal of tumor and these methods have remained the same over the past few decades (Mukherjee et al., 2011). The treatments mentioned above usually include a considerable risk associated with the toxicity and immunosuppression of the non-cancerous cells and the cancer cells. Of the many challenges involved in the treatment of OSCC, one of the main concern includes transportation of drugs specifically to the target region. Also, the cancer stem cells (CSCs), which are a part of the population, remains dormant and escapes most of the treatment. Chemoresistance is also an issue as the cancer cells develop resistance against the drugs. These limitations result in the cancer treatment being less efficient. Thus, targeted cancer therapy is the correct approach for cancer treatment. This can be achieved by the use of delivery agents loaded with the required drug and designed to specifically target the cancer cells with the help of specific markers. Nanoparticles can be used as delivery agents due to their small size and ability to carry the desired molecular cargo (therapeutic drugs) and this branch of treatment is called Nanomedicine. The drug delivered to the cancer site by utilizing Nano-delivery methods is observed to be in high concentration in that area and do not affect the surrounding cells. Nanomedicine is a technology already in use and provides promising results in targeted cancer therapy. Improvements in Nanomedicine can be of a great aid in the fight against cancer due to their stability and specificity in cancer treatment.

ORAL CANCER

Oral Squamous Cell Carcinoma (OSCC) is one of the most frequently observed malignancies found in patients with head and neck cancers. OSCC is a type of oral cancer where the oral epithelial cells are damaged due to the accumulation of multiple genetic mutations (Calcaterra et al., 1995). In India, more than 130,000 people develop OSCC in a year and this is due to the consumption of tobacco in the form of gutka, betel quid, snuff and mishri (Thomas et al., 1993). The consumption of areca nut by most Asians poses a potential risk for oral cancer (Gupta et al., 2002) (Warnakulasuriya et al., 2002). These chronic carcinogens cause infections and destroy the mucosal lining of the oral cavity resulting in OSCC (Gillenwater et al., 2006). Tobacco is the leading cause of OSCC with the incidence rate being more than 90% and when consumed along with alcohol/chewing tobacco, the rate of occurrence is increased by many folds (Jordan et al., 1997). Thus, non-smokers are less likely to develop OSCC when compared to smokers with the occurrence being 4-7 times more in smokers (Ko et al., 1995). Other than tobacco, immunosuppressed patients (HIV) are also at the risk of developing OSCC (Petersen et al., 2009) (Jones et al., 2008). Also, Human Papilloma

Virus (HPV) results in viral infections leading to OSCC (Huang et al., 2008). The occurrence is more in males than in females with the mortality rate also being higher in males (Su et al., 2007) (Chen et al., 2002). The 5-year mortality rate of OSCC patients is 50% worldwide (Kantola et al., 2000) and treatments mostly include chemotherapy and radiation therapy. These treatment methods are less efficient and also have a higher risk of damaging the surrounding cells. The chances of cancer recurrence in patients undergoing chemotherapy/radiation therapy increases in about 18-76% of cases. The lack of early detection leads to complication in patients, and thus treatment becomes challenging and less effective (Shah et al., 1995). Researchers and clinicians opinethat OSCC can be reduced by changing lifestyle and educating people about the issues related to oral cancer and minimizing the use of carcinogenic substances like tobacco which plays an important role in OSCC occurrence.

CHALLENGES AND LIMITATIONS IN OSCC TREATMENT

Although expert clinicians can easily examine oral cavity, up to 50% of oral cancer is not detectable in the early stages of cancer, making it difficult to decide the proper course of treatment. (Yu et al., 2008). Primary stage detection may help to decrease the death rate in oral cancer and the survival rate of 90% of the oral cancer patients is less than 5 years (Popovtzer et al., 2008). Early-stage screening of oral cancer is usually performed by two different approaches, one is a screening program and the second is a sensitive early diagnostic tool for asymptomatic patients. Though the National Cancer Institute's SEER program in USA generates information on the cancer affected population, stages of cancer and mortality rate, it has not been able to derive data on early diagnosis of OSCC (Ries et al., 2008).

OSCC treatments currently in use are chemotherapy, radiation therapy, surgical removal, antibody-based therapy and combined therapies. The method of treatment for OSCC depends on the stages of cancer (Shah et al., 1995) and the current treatment protocols have certain limitations. Surgically removing the tumor is highly risky due to the presence of several other intricately associated tissues in the vicinity of the tumor site. Sometimes even after surgery, some of the cancer residues remain, which may contain the cancer stem cells and in future it can lead to recurrence and metastasis of the cancer. Radiation therapy is another method for treating OSCC, but it has high failure rates for advanced tumors. Additionally, there is a risk of toxicity to the normal cells and thus it may lead to the damage of the oral cavity and the cells surrounding it. Chemotherapy for OSCC patients is usually done in combination with radiation therapy. Also, chemotherapy is not specific only to the tumor cells and hence damage to the surrounding cells is observed along with the cancer cells. Chemotherapy is used along with radiation therapy only in stages III or IV and is more effective when done as a combinatorial treatment (Scully et al, 2013; Shah et al., 1995). Cisplatin, Docetaxel (DTX), Cetuximab, Paclitaxel, Fluorouracil and Methotrexate are few of the chemotherapeutic drugs used for OSCC treatment (Adelstein et al., 2003; Agüeros et al., 2009; Baselga et al., 2005; Bonner et al., 2006; Haddad et al., 2009; Scully, 2013; Vermorken et al., 2007a,b, 2008). Chemotherapy and antibody blocking therapy are effective when used with radiation therapy for organ preservation (Bonner et al., 2006; Myers et al., 2003). These chemotherapeutic drugs can be orally taken and most patients prefer oral admission as it is easier and the cells in the mouth are in contact with these drugs for more time when taken orally (Terwogt et al., 1999). The limitations of these orally administered drugs are poor absorption and also dissolve poorly in water (Agüeros et al., 2009; Devalapally et al., 2007). Another method for drug intake is intravenous administration and absorption through the gastrointestinal tract. In this method, more bioavailability is observed but it has the risk of non-specific cytotoxicity that affects the normal cells along with cancer cells (Kruijtzer et al., 2002). Cancer patients have a lot of complications involving both the side effects of treatment or disease or due to some other reasons which makes the treatment even more complex. OSCC patients have complications mostly due to the use of chemotherapy/radiation therapy which slows or stops the rate of fast-growing cells. The normal cells lining the inner region of the human oral cavity are rapidly dividing and these cells can be damaged by the treatment. Thus, the repairing ability of the oral cavity cells is greatly reduced. Similarly, radiation therapy can directly cause degradation of oral tissues, salivary glands and bones. Many bacteria are present in the oral cavity and there is a balance between the beneficial and harmful bacteria. Chemo/ radiation therapy disrupts this balance and also kills many beneficial bacteria. These alterations result in infections and sores in the oral cavity and thus cause changes in taste and pain. These result in malnutrition, dehydration and other such problems (Scully et al., 2013). These limitations and complications can be overcome by the use of new strategies for the targeted treatment of the OSCC. The technique of interest here is the delivery of therapeutic agents *via* nanoparticles, which is gaining importance in the treatment of cancer patients.

NANOTECHNOLOGY

Nanotechnology is the science that refers to the manipulation of materials at the atomic level. (Seigneuric et al., 2010). Nanotechnology was first explained by the Nobel laureate Richard Feynman in his seminal lecture as, "There is plenty of room at the bottom" in 1959 (Moghimi et al., 2006). It is a multidisciplinary dynamic approach using materials as designs and is an interdisciplinary area including the combination of chemistry, physics, engineering, medicine and biology. (Sahoo et al., 2007). Nano research is related to fundamental cell and molecular biology and manipulated engineered materials like the subatomic particles in the biological system. It is based on particles manipulation *via t*op-up and bottom down approaches. A very interesting side of nanotechnology is the nanoscience-based investigations that are performed at the nano level. Nanotechnology contributes to an understanding of the intra molecular approaches in biology. The National Cancer Institute (NCI)/ National Institute of Health (NIH) of the United States had accepted that nanotechnology offers an extensive domain that creates a convenient approach for cancer investigation and treatment. Thus, it opens up new avenues in cancer diagnosis, treatment and prevention (Pridgen et al., 2007).

NANOMEDICINE

Nanomedicine is a great promising area of nanotechnology. Nanomedicine aims to clinically screen samples as early as possible, to treat cancer in an effective manner with minimal toxicity and high target efficiency (Caruthers et al., 2007; Shaffer et al., 2005). Last few decades of nano research focused on the development of effective and efficient drug transport system (e.g., micelles, gelatin nanoparticles and liposomes) which could play a crucial role in nanomedicine research. Recent nanoscience development involves innovative platforms based on gold nanoparticles, Quantum Dots (QDs), carbon nanotubes and paramagnetic nanoparticles and other domains which are based on lipid nanomaterials. Some nano systems are also used for nano therapy, such as nanoliposomes, dendrimers, nanotubes and QDs. In the case of cancer, detection tool development peruses gold nanoparticles and surface-enhanced Raman spectroscopy (SERS) nanoparticles show more promising activity with low toxicity (Paciotti et al., 2006; Cai et al., 2008). Currently, Nanotech based biochip platforms are used for molecular diagnostics of DNA, RNA and protein identification. Nanomedicine contributes to solve several medical complications by utilizing new techniques and innovative approaches (Caruthers et al., 2007; Freitas et al, 2005a,b). Nanomedicine has the potential to change the bio-distribution of drug and pharmacokinetics. The development of the nanomedicine field is more effective and promising due to the dynamics involved in understanding the role of drug delivery, disease screening, etc., (Manmode et al., 2009; Manohar et al., 2011; Moghimi et al., 2005; Mohanraj et al., 2006). Nanomedicine is one of the leading approaches which can contribute towards the invention of personalized medicines.

CANCER NANOTECHNOLOGY

Cancer Nanotechnology research constructs a dynamic platform to overcome several unsolved cancer biology related problems. Analysis based on targeted approaches are directed so that the therapeutic agent can kill cancer cells specifically with low toxicity to normal cells. Scientists are developing an agent which can aid in cancer diagnosis, prevention and recovery. Targeted drug and gene delivery innovated by Osaka University in Japan (Yamada et al., 2003), Southwest Research Institute (SwRI), Texas, have devised nano capsules that can carry antibody, vaccine and drug to a specific site with minimal side effects (Saravana et al., 2006; Sha et al., 2007). Nanoparticles have a double signature role, one, it works as a drug carrier, and the other absorbs a different wavelength of light. When there is application of specific wave length, nanoparticles are heated up and kill temperature sensitive cancer cells. Nanoparticles are ultra-small size, and because of that, they can even enter parts of the body like tiny small capillary vessels escaping phagocytosis and in tissue gaps in targeted sites. Nanoparticles are capable of targeting tumor actively and passively and these characteristics of nanoparticles makes it an innovative option for cancer detection, imaging and prevention (Calixto et al., 2014; Sindura et al., 2013). As a newly emerging field, cancer nanotechnology has created a signature in advanced cancer screening and treatment. The innovative engineering of material science at the nanoscale level helps to develop highly effective cancer treatments.

NANOTECHNOLOGY AND OSCC

OSCC affects a large population and is the cause of a high rate of mortality and morbidity worldwide. Newly emerging scientific research investigations are involved in identifying an early diagnosis marker for OSCC. Nanotechnology is an efficient platform for OSCC research in developing molecular imaging, primary level screening and impactful specific treatment. Worldwide scientific research focuses on innovative advanced drug delivery systems and early detection tools for OSCC.

NANOTECHNOLOGY IN OSCC DIAGNOSIS

The main advantage of using nanoparticles in OSCC diagnosis or treatment is their microscopic size and flexibility. They utilize the rapid proliferation, leaky tumor vasculature and specific cell surface antigen expression of the cancer cells to their advantage for the diagnosis (Bhandare et al., 2014). Many nano-diagnostic tools originated earlier to detect OSCC, such as cantilevers, gold nanoparticles, nano shells, nanopores, nanotubes, and QDs. Nanoscale cantilevers are elastic beams applied to attract cancer-specific biomolecules and bind to these specific biomolecules. (Liu et al., 2013; Mubben et al., 2010). Carbon rods termed nanotubes are used to detect defective genes and localize their location.

Similarly, nanopores provide highly efficient sequencing as it allows the DNA to pass through the minute holes in them (one strand at a time). QDs are semiconductor fluorescent nanocrystals made of cadmium-selenide. These attach to the proteins associated with cancer and glow brightly under UV thus identifying the location of the tumors (Bhardwaj et al., 2013). Tumor biomarkers that can detect cancer early are being developed and hence newer strategies using nanotechnology to identify these markers in the saliva (for OSCC) and other body fluids are also been investigated (Omar et al., 2015). Photoluminescent nanoparticles help to differentiate the normal cells from that of the cancer cells. The nanoparticles can detect tumor because they release specific biomarker molecules such as peptides when they attach to the tumor. Nanoparticles carry several peptides, and hence when they attach to the tumor, they release a high concentration of these peptides, making cancer detection easier and thus cancer can be detected at a very early stage. Likewise, QDs and MRI hold an application for imaging tumor (Hatziantoniou et al., 2006; Virupakshappa et al., 2012). Exosomes are small extracellular vesicles that are elevated in cancer conditions and can also act as biomarkers for detection. Exosomes are sources of proteomic and genomic markers for cancer investigations. . The presence of these exosomes can be determined using atomic force microscopy that employs nanoparticles (Gau et al., 2007). Salivary biomarkers can be detected using the Oral fluid nano sensor test (OFNASET) method, where eight markers can be detected within 15 minutes (Eifler et al., 2011; Vogell et al., 2013; Wei et al., 2011). Thus, many such nanotechnological methods are being used or investigated to detect and localize tumor in the patients.

NANOTECHNOLOGY IN OSCC TREATMENT

The OSCC patients are treated with certain chemotherapy drugs which are used alone or in combinations. The local drug delivery usually has limitations such as improper absorption of drugs by the oral tissues, the reduced availability of drugs for patients and the limited potential for drug absorption etc., (Dodla et al., 2013). Cytotoxicity to normal cells and non-specific targeting of the cancer cells are the other main limitations (Lida et al., 2013). Nanotechnology to treat OSCC patientshas great advantage due to effective drug loading, transport, controlled drug release, specificity to cancer cells and non-toxicity to normal cells. The use of nanoparticles increases stability and controls targeted drug delivery, which is generally a problem faced in other procedures. The nanoparticles delivery also ensures the uniform concentration of the drugs at the site of lesions and extravasation of drugs is facilitated into the target site by reducing the toxicity to normal cells (Brannon-Peppas et al., 2012; Brewer et al., 2011; Mahapatro et al., 2011). Another advantage is the biocompatibility and biodistribution of nanoparticles, resulting in highly efficient drug delivery (Elbayoumi et al., 2010). The commonly used nanoparticles for drug delivery are liposomes, polymeric nanoparticles, carbon nanotubes, dendrimers, magnetic nanoparticles and gold particles (Jain et al., 2010; Kapse-Mistry et al., 2014; Khan et al., 2014; Paciotti et al., 2004; Tang et al., 2010). Antibodies are also utilized against cancer cells for treatment. Epidermal Growth Factor Receptor (EGFR) is present in all the epithelial cells and cancers of epithelial cells have overexpressed EGFR. Thus, anti-EGFR antibody-conjugated nanorods can specifically bind to the cancer cells (El-Sayed et al., 2006) and the malignant cells can be easily differentiated from the non-malignant cells (Huang et al., 2006). The method includes exposing the cells to an undistorted red laser at 800nm. Earlier tests have shown that only about 50%

of the laser energy is required for degrading the malignant cells. This provides the information for effective photothermal treatment of cancer cells. These methods also help in the easy diagnosis of the OSCC. (El-Sayed et al., 2006; Huang et al., 2007) AuNPs (gold nanoparticles) manage cancer therapy in patients as they uptake light and produce heat for plasmonic photothermal treatment (PPTT). The nanoparticles are designed accordingly to be tuned over the visible and NIR (near-infrared light) region. The nanoparticles are tuned over 650-1000 nm as the penetration at this wavelength is maximal for the human cells (Cui et al., 2011; Sukhija et al., 2015). Gold particles hold demand for the transport of nucleic acids, photothermal and radiotherapy drug delivery agents. High radiation dosage to the cancer cells adopting these gold particle approaches absorbs sufficient X-rays. Thus, once the gold particles are localized into tumor, they concentrate the radiations towards the cancer cells alone (El-Sayed et al., 2006; Huang et al., 2006). The benefits of tuning up the nanoparticles to our interest results in high biocompatibility and less cytotoxicity. Nanoshells are another method for treating OSCC patients wherein tiny beads could specifically target and accumulate in the cancer cells (James et al., 2007). Thus, gold nanoshells also helps in increased absorption of radiation in the cancer cells, thus limiting their survival in the patients (Liu et al., 2010).

NANO-BASED DRUG DELIVERY FOR OSCC

Applications of nanotechnology-based drug delivery system renders more stability and specificity to deliver the drugs to the target site (Reddy et al., 2015). Researchers are developing nanoparticles, including liposomes, hydrogels, polymeric micelles, dendrimers, nanospheres, nano capsules and nanotubes (Cui et al., 2011; Paciotti et al., 2006; Park et al., 2004; Praetorius et al., 2007). Therapeutic drugs can be loaded into the nanoparticles and can act as the drug delivery agents to the cancer cells (Peer et al., 2007). Liposomes are microscopic particles artificially made to act as nano-vectors (Park et al., 2002). They are spherical, can be unilamellar or multi-lamellar and are basically made up of lipids surrounding a water core. Liposomes are promising drug carriers due to their size, biocompatibility, ease of preparation and hydrophobicity. These liposomes can be coated with PEG (Polyethylene glycol) to increase their circulation time in the blood for more absorption. These are the most widely used drug delivery agents due to their specificity to the target, less cellular toxicity to the normal cells and also delivers the chemotherapy drugs to the target sites precisely(Calixto et al., 2014; De Lima et al., 2001; Lian et al., 2001; Park et al., 2002). Hydrogel is a mesh of Hydrophilic polymer chains dispersed in water, capable of delivering drugs to the target site *via* the gaps in the mesh. They swell and can easily carry loads of therapeutic drugs (Bahram et al., 2014). The main advantage of hydrogels is the rapid release of the drug content to the target sites (Salamat-Miller et al., 2005). Thus, they release drugs in the oral cavity before being washed away by the salivary enzymes. Due to their close interaction with the salivary glycoproteins, hydrogels are usually administered orally and are effective in treating OSCC (Gao et al., 2011; Hao et al., 2009; Konishi et al., 2005; Tang-na et al., 2009; Tauro et al., 2005). Biodegradable polymers such as Poly (D, L, lactide-co-glycolide) (PLGA) and PEG are used for the production of theranostic polymer nanoparticles (Vijayakumar et al., 2013). Controlled release of drugs can be achieved by using nanotechnology. ReGel is one example of such polymer-based drug delivery (Zentner et al., 2001). The antitumor effect of herpes simplex virus thymidine kinase loaded PEG on the OSCC cells is being used to treat cancer. Nanoparticle mediated HSV-tk treatment is another efficient way of treating OSCC (Yu et al., 2008b). Liquid crystal is a material present in the mesophase (a phase between solid and liquid) and it can be designed to manipulate the amount of drug to be released and can reduce the toxicity of the released drugs (Formariz et al., 2005). The drugs are supplemented to the liquid crystal along with the help of substances like glycerides (Hosmer et al., 2012). Polyphosphate coated magnetic nanoparticles (MNPs) can also be used for the delivery of drugs specifically and efficiently to OSCC patients (Candido et al., 2014). A nanostructured lipid carrier (NLC) is a new nanodevice used for drug delivery.

Table 1.

Carriers for Drug Delivery	Advantages	Disadvantages	References
Polymeric nanoparticles	Biodegradable and biocompatible Suitable for controlled and sustained drugs release with increased therapeutic effeacy and reduced side effects	Dicult to handle due to particle-particle aggregation Cytotoxic after internalization into cells Not suitable for the release of proteins including antibodies Associated with an immune response or local toxicity upon degradation	(Jawahar et al., 2012) (Sim et al., 2011) (Rizvi et al., 2018) (Kulkarni et al., 2013) (Hoshyar et al., 2016)
Inorganic nanoparticles	Target can be site specific by attaching the ligand to the nanoparticle (e.g., magnetic nanoparticles) Higher photostability compared to organic dyes	Toxicity Limited e_ective delivery due to limited penetration depth for photothermal therapy Cannot deliver bio macromolecules (e.g., proteins)	(Huang et al., 2011) (Subramani et al., 2012) (Sato et al., 2016)
Nanolipids	Highly stable Provide controlled release of drugs to protect them from chemical degradation Encapsulate and deliver drugs with low aqueous solubility Able to penetrate deeply into tumors Suitable for local delivery of anticancer drugs	Crystalline structure provides limited space to accommodate drugs Solid lipid nanoparticles (SLNs) show initial burst drug release Aggregation or gelling of nanostructured lipid carriers (NLCs) during storage Associated with immune response	(Sim et al., 2011) (Ghasemiyeh et al., 2018) (Khosa et al., 2018) (Calixto et al., 2014) (Sun et al., 2012)
Hydrogels	Injectable to a specific site Do not dissolve in water at physiological temperature and pH Maintain their structural integrity and elasticity even after retaining large amounts of water	Poor mechanical properties Difficult to handle Expensive Initial burst	(Coelho et al., 2010) (Singh et al., 2014)

It has a significant advantage over other methods due to the presence of a liquid-lipid nano-compartment. More drugs can be carried and released as there is no crystallization of lipids with solid (Lin et al., 2010). The advantages and disadvantages of each carrier has been summarized in the table.

Clinical Trials of Nanomedicine for OSCC

Nanotechnology-based drug delivery system shows excellent efficiency in treating OSCC, which guarantees less cytotoxicity, more specificity and controlled release of the drug. A study was performed on two different cell lines (malignant and non-malignant) which were selectively targeted using plasmonic photothermal therapy (PPTT), where a laser at 442 nm (visible region) resulted in the efficient killing of the malignant cell lines at much lower energy, compared to the non-malignant cell lines (El-Sayed et al., 2006; Huang et al., 2006). Also, radioactive material-coated nanoparticles are under trial to destroy tumor when placed nearby or within the target site (Mousa et al., 2011; Shetty et al., 2013). NIR photothermal therapy with gold nanoshells (Auralase) is under human trial in refractory head and neck cancers.

A study has reported applying gold nanoparticles to enhance radiation therapy by sensitizing the resistant cancer cells in mouse head and neck squamous cell cancer models (Kang et al., 2010). A study conducted on human oral cancer cells demonstrated the efficacy of liposomal mediated aluminum phthalocyanine chloride-based photodynamic therapy in inhibiting the phosphatidylinositol, 3-kinase/Akt/mammalian (p13K/Akt/mTOR) signaling pathway (Velloso et al., 2012) (Figueiró Longo et al., 2012). Similarly, the application of liposomes has been exploited as carriers for several drugs such as all-trans-retinoic acid (ATRA), doxorubicin, gefitinib, cetuximab, tirapazamine, etc., Besides, treatment with liposomal cisplatin reportedly reduced renal and hematological toxicity of advanced OSCC (Calixto et al., 2014; Park et al., 2008). The rate of cisplatin release modulated using an acrylic hydrogel known as p9, might be a promising platform for chemotherapy of OSCC (Casolaro et al., 2009) (Fang et al., 2011). ReGel a polymer-based delivery system has the structure as PLGA-PEG-PLGA (Zentner et al., 2001). Oncogel is a type of ReGel with Paclitaxel used for the delivery of paclitaxel to the cancer cells. Oncogel is successfully used for OSCC treatment as the drug is released for six weeks to the tumor and the microenvironment with this method (Elstad et al., 2009; Marupudi et al., 2007; Zeng et al., 2012). Curcumin and genistein are poorly accessible molecules that can be delivered orally with the help of NLC devices with promising results (Aditya et al., 2013) (Zlotogorski et al., 2013). Two drugs, namely Doxil (doxorubicin encapsulated liposomes) and Abraxane (nanoparticle albumin-bound paclitaxel) have been shown to have a wide range of anti-tumor activity against a variety of cancers including OSCC, and have been approved by FDA (Nagahara et al., 2007; Tang et al., 2010). Recently a few other drugs have also been approved for the treatment of different cancer types (Bedikian et al., 2011). Nano drugs approval consumes a lot of time and is a slow process but with promising results in the treatment of various cancers, such as OSCC.

SAFETY ISSUES OF NANOTECHNOLOGY

Though all of the advantages in nanotechnology have been highlighted, it has few drawbacks, especially safety. Therefore, it must be done with utmost care without causing harm to the researchers and the clinicians. Due to the advancements in the field of nanotechnology, the toxicity associated with nanoparticles can be manipulated effectively by several functionalization methods. Nanomaterials have large surfaces that have high loading capability. It also consists of a charged surface with high reactivity that plays a role in human body absorption *via* skin, lung and digestive tract. In this process, nanomaterials are accumulated in different parts of the body *via* the blood system. This deposition of material causes inflammation in the lungs and causes damage to the cells Nanoparticles can react with nucleic acids (DNA, RNA) and proteins and other intracellular components, and thus contribute to mutations (Upadhyay et al., 2013). Another safety concern is that the particles are non-biodegradable and may deposit in several organs like the kidney and liver and cause damage which requires further investigation as this is a relatively new field. Because of such intricacies, the use of nanomedicine as an alternative cancer treatment requires further assessment. As such, it could be challenging to establish the rules and regulations for nanotechnology safety assessments. Dynamic and innovative nanomedcine requires more pharmacokinetic and toxicokinetic studies for its daily life applications. Thus, nanotechnology can create a new history in the health care industry, if nanomedicine is adequately used with efficient safety management protocols.

Future Perspectives

Nanotechnology has the ability to provide challenges to the traditional health care system. It has paved way for more innovative ways of screening and prevention of OSCC. Furthermore, nanotechnology opens a new platform for developing personalized medicines, and it is demonstrating more effectiveness in the delivery of therapeutic drugs and gene therapy. It may play a vital role in the innovation of advanced diagnostic tools for clinical checkup and modern therapeutics like nanodevices which include photo-thermal and magneto-thermal probes, vectors for drug and gene delivery and radiation inducers. OSCC markers investigation is currently based on bioinformatics and proteomics, but the applications of nanodevices are far more sensitive and efficient when compared with them. Recent OSCC therapies face several challenges which are (1) non-specific anti-cancer agents, (2) identifying the right amount of drug that reaches the target site, (3) intolerable cytotoxicity of nanomedicine, (4) few ways to observe therapeutic responses and (5) resistance to multiple drugs (Ehdaie et al., 2007). New innovative approaches are required to detect the cells in micro-metastasis levels and to kill the tumor cell completely. The multifunctional role of nanomaterials as a targeting and therapeutic agent against OSCC is welcoming and can assist to alleviate the sufferings of the patients. It helps chemotherapeutic drugs to reach the specific site of cancer and as a result, it increases the efficiency of treatment *via* a low dose of the drug with better impact.

Nanodevice is utilized for screening and imaging and specific targeting of the drugs. Liposomal-based anticancer drug delivery needs more investigation for industrial-level production. In future, additional research necessitates determining the practical therapeutic effect of curcumin-loaded nanostructured lipid carriers (NLCs) for OSCC treatment. The ATRA-loaded NLCs show promising activity in OSCC treatment. (Chinsriwongkul et al., 2012; Liu et al., 2013, 2014; Wang et al., 2013). Few nanomedicines have the ability to deliver drug to different parts of the body with high specificity as demonstrated by the National Cancer Institute USA manufacture unit. (Hull et al., 2014). This technology using nanoparticles can contribute to developing a drug that will have the property to minimize the side effects (Fakruddin et al., 2012). The designed nano-base robot has complete control over drug delivery and its activity. Dynamic functionality is the crucial property of nanoparticles that helps to overcome all other limitations of traditional treatment approaches. Nanoparticle conjugated strategies play a role in targeting ligands, imaging labels, therapeutic drugs and molecular therapy in OSCC. The innovative way for OSCC treatment is to develop nanomedicines on a molecular marker-based specific therapy. (Kumar et al., 2012a, b; Shim et al., 2010; Sumer et al., 2008). The nanotechnology-based early detection approach is very impactful because of its capability to detect OSCC at an early stages (Von Maltzahn et al., 2009) using photothermal methods based on gold nanorods to cure cancer in *in vivo* model. In future, nanomedicine can play a vital role towards the prevention of OSCC at the cellular level.

CONCLUSION

The development of nanotechnology and engineered multifunctional nanoparticles contribute to the innovation of futuristic early screening tool and treatment method for OSCC. Different *in vitro* and *in vivo* investigations has shown that nanotechnology is more promising for overcoming several challenges in OSCC diagnosis and therapy. A multifunctional nanotechnology-based smart device is more sensitive and specific for OSCC diagnosis. Scientific research on applied nanotechnology in OSCC treatment is very impactful. It involves combination of nanotechnology-with proteomic or genomic based research for cancer biomarkers investigation. Some nano formulated medicines are in Phase I and II clinical trials. Traditional side effects of chemotherapy method can be silently replaced by novel nanotechnology-based active or passive targeting therapeutic methods. As a result, it can influence the survival rate of OSCC patients. Nanotechnology is still an advancing research area that necessitates additional research for developing effective diagnostics tool and therapeutic methods to alleviate the sufferings of OSCC patients.

REFERENCES

Adelstein, D. J., Li, Y., Adams, G. L., Wagner, Jr., H., Kish, J. A., Ensley, J. F., Schuller, D. E., Forastiere, A. A., 2003. An intergroup phase III comparison of standard radiation therapy and two schedules of concurrent chemoradiotherapy in patients with unresectable squamous cell head and neck cancer. *J. Clin. Oncol.* 21 (1), 92–98.

Aditya, N., Shim, M., Lee, I., Lee, Y., Im, M. H., Ko, S., 2013. Curcumin and genistein coloaded nanostructured lipid carriers: *in vitro* digestion and antiprostate cancer activity. *J. Agr. Food Chem.* 61, 1878–1883.

Agüeros, M., Ruiz-Gatón, L., Vauthier, C., Bouchemal, K., Espuelas, S., Ponchel, G., Irache, J. M., 2009. Combined hydroxypropyl-β-cyclodextrin and poly (anhydride) nanoparticles improve the oral permeability of paclitaxel. *Eur. J. Pharm. Sci.* 38 (4), 405–413.

Agüeros, M., Ruiz-Gatón, L., Vauthier, C., Bouchemal, K., Espuelas, S., Ponchel, G., Irache, J. M., 2009. Combined hydroxypropyl-β-cyclodextrin and poly(anhydride) nanoparticles improve the oral permeability of paclitaxel. *Eur. J. Pharm. Sci.* 38 (4), 405–413.

Bahram, M., Hoseinzadeh, F., Farhadi, K., Saadat, M., Najafi-Moghaddam, P., Afkhami, A., 2014. Synthesis of gold nanoparticles using pH-sensitive hydrogel and its application for colorimetric determination of acetaminophen, ascorbic acid and folic acid. *Colloids Surf.* 441, 517–524.

Baselga, J., Trigo, J. M., Bourhis, J., Tortochaux, J., Cortés-Funes, H., Hitt, R., Gascón, P., Amellal, N., Harstrick, A., Eckardt, A., 2005. Phase II multicenter study of the antiepidermal growth factor receptor monoclonal antibody cetuximab in combination with platinum-based chemotherapy in patients with platinum-refractory metastatic and/or recurrent squamous cell carcinoma of the head and neck. *J. Clin. Oncol.* 23 (24), 5568–5577.

Bedikian, A. Y., Silverman, J. A., Papadopoulos, N. E., Kim, K. B., Hagey, A. E., Vardeleon, A., Hwu, W. J., Homzi, J., Davies, M., Hwu, P., 2011. Pharmacokinetics and safety of Marqibo (vincristine sulfate liposomes injection) in cancer patients with impaired liver function. *J. Clin. Pharmacol.* 51, 1205–1212.

Bhandare, N., Narayana, A., 2014. Applications of nanotechnology in cancer. A literature review of imaging and treatment. *J. Nucl. Med. Radat. Ther.* 5 (4), 195.

Bhardwaj, A., Misuriya, A., Maroli, S., Manjula, S., Singh, A. K., 2013. Nanotechnology in dentistry: present and future. *J. Int. Oral. Health 6* (1), 121–126.

Bonner, J. A., Harari, P. M., Giralt, J., Azarnia, N., Shin, D. M., Cohen, R. B., Jones, C. U., Sur, R., Raben, D., Jassem, J., Ove, R., Kies, M. S., Baselga, J., Youssoufian, H., Amellal, N., Rowinsky, E. K., Ang, K. K., 2006. Radiotherapy plus cetuximab for squamous-cell carcinoma of the head and neck. *N. Engl. J. Med.* 354 (6), 567–578.

Bonner, J. A., Harari, P. M., Giralt, J., Azarnia, N., Shin, D. M., Cohen, R. B., Jones, C. U., Sur, R., Raben, D., Jassem, J., Ove, R., Kies, M. S., Baselga, J., Youssoufian, H., Amellal, N., Rowinsky, E. K., Ang, K. K., 2006. Radiotherapy plus cetuximab for squamous-cell carcinoma of the head and neck. *N. Engl. J. Med.* 354 (6), 567–578.

Brannon-Peppas, L., Blanchette, J. O., 2012. Nanoparticle and targeted systems for cancer therapy. *Adv. Drug. Deliv. Rev.* 64, 206–212.

Brewer, E., Coleman, J., Lowman, A., 2011. Emerging technologies of polymeric nanoparticles in cancer drug delivery. *J. Nanomater.*

Cai, W., Gao, T., Hong, H., et al., 2008. Applications of gold nanoparticles in cancer nanotechnology. *Nanotechnol. Sci. Appl.* 1, 17–32.

Calcaterra TC, Juillard GJ. Oral cavity and hypopharynx-head and neck cancer. In: Haskell CM, Berek JS, editors. *Cancer treatment.* Philadelphia: WB Saunders Co; 1995. pp. 726–32.

Calixto, G., Bernegossi, J., Fonseca-Santos, B., Chorilli, M., 2014. Nanotechnology-based drug delivery systems for treatment of oral cancer—a review. *Int. J. Nanomed.* 9, 3719–3735.

Calixto, G., Bernegossi, J., Fonseca-Santos, B., Chorilli, M., 2014. Nanotechnology-based drug delivery systems for treatment of oral cancer—a review. *Int. J. Nanomed.* 9, 3719–3735.

Calixto, G., Bernegossi, J., Fonseca-Santos, B., Chorilli, M., 2014. Nanotechnology-based drug delivery systems for treatment of oral cancer—a review. *Int. J. Nanomed.* 9, 3719–3735.

Calixto, G.; Bernegossi, J.; Fonseca-Santos, B.; Chorilli, M. Nanotechnology-based drug delivery systems for treatment of oral cancer: A review. *Int. J. Nanomed.* 2014, 9, 3719–3735.

Candido, N., Calmon, M. d. F., Taboga, S. R, Bonilha, J. L., Dos Santos, M., Lima, E. C. d. O., Sousa, C., Lacava, Z. G. M., Rahal, P., 2014. High efficacy in hyperthermia-associated with polyphosphate magnetic nanoparticles for oral cancer treatment. *J. Nanomed. Nanotechnol.* 5, 1–11.

Caruthers, S. D., Wickline, S. A., Lanza, G. M., 2007. Nanotechnological applications in medicine. *Curr. Opin. Biotechnol.* 18 (1), 26–30.

Caruthers, S. D., Wickline, S. A., Lanza, G. M., 2007. Nanotechnological applications in medicine. *Curr. Opin. Biotechnol.* 18 (1), 26–30.

Casolaro, M., Cini, R., Del Bello, B., Ferrali, M., Maellaro, E., 2009. Cisplatin/hydrogel complex in cancer therapy. *Biomacromolecules* 10 (4), 944–949. doi: 10.1021/bm8014939.

Chen CJ, You SL, Lin LH, Hsu WL, Yang YW. Cancer epidemiology and control in Taiwan: a brief review. *Jpn J Cancer Res.* 2002; 32 Suppl: S66–S81.

Chinsriwongkul, A., Chareanputtakhun, P., Ngawhirunpat, T., Rojanarata, T., Sila-On, W., Ruktanonchai, U., Opanasopit, P., 2012. Nanostructured lipid carriers (NLC) for parenteral delivery of an anticancer drug. *AAPS PharmSciTech* 13, 150–158.

Coelho, J. F.; Ferreira, P. C.; Alves, P.; Cordeiro, R.; Fonseca, A. C.; Góis, J. R.; Gil, M. H. Drug delivery systems: Advanced technologies potentially applicable in personalized treatments. *EPMA J.* 2010, 1, 164–209.

Cui, D., Huang, P., Zhang, C., Ozkan, C. S., Pan, B., Xu, P., 2011. Dendrimer-modified gold nanorods as efficient controlled gene delivery system under near-infrared light irradiation. *J. Control. Release* 152 (Suppl. 1), e137–e139.

Cui, D., Huang, P., Zhang, C., Ozkan, C. S., Pan, B., Xu, P., 2011. Dendrimer-modified gold nanorods as efficient controlled gene delivery system under near-infrared light irradiation. *J. Control. Release* 152 (Suppl. 1), e137–e139.

De Lima, M. C. P., Simões, S., Pires, P., Faneca, H., Düzgüneş, N., 2001. Cationic lipid–DNA complexes in gene delivery: from biophysics to biological applications. *Adv. Drug Deliv. Rev.* 47, 277–294.

Devalapally, H., Chakilam, A., Amiji, M. M., 2007. Role of nanotechnology in pharmaceutical product development. *J. Pharm. Sci.* 96 (10), 2547–2565.

Dodla, S., Velmurugan, S., 2013. Buccal penetration enhancers: an overview. *Asian J. Pharm. Clin. Res.* 6, 39–47.

Ehdaie, B., 2007. Application of nanotechnology in cancer research: review of progress in the National Cancer Institute's Alliance for Nanotechnology. *Int. J. Biol. Sci.* 3 (2), 108.

Eifler, A. C., Thaxton, C. S., 2011. Nanoparticle therapeutics: FDA approval, clinical trials, regulatory pathways, and case study. *Methods Mol. Biol.* 726, 325–338.

Elbayoumi, T. A., 2010. Nano drug-delivery systems in cancer therapy: gains, pitfalls and considerations in DMPK and PD. *Ther. Deliv.* 1 (2), 215–219.

El-Sayed, I. H., Huang, X., El-Sayed, M. A., 2006. Selective laser photothermal therapy of epithelial carcinoma using anti-EGFR antibody conjugated gold nanoparticles. *Cancer Lett.* 239 (1), 129–135.

El-Sayed, I. H., Huang, X., El-Sayed, M. A., 2006. Selective laser photothermal therapy of epithelial carcinoma using anti-EGFR antibody conjugated gold nanoparticles. *Cancer Lett.* 239 (1), 129–135.

El-Sayed, I. H., Huang, X., El-Sayed, M. A., 2006. Selective laser photothermal therapy of epithelial carcinoma using anti-EGFR antibody conjugated gold nanoparticles. *Cancer Lett.* 239 (1), 129–135.

El-Sayed, I.H., Huang, X., El-Sayed, M.A., 2006. Selective laser photothermal therapy of epithelial carcinoma using anti-EGFR antibody conjugated gold nanoparticles. *Cancer Lett.* 239 (1), 129–135.

Elstad, N. L., Fowers, K. D., 2009. OncoGel (ReGel/paclitaxel)—clinical applications for a novel paclitaxel delivery system. *Adv. Drug Deliv. Rev.* 61 (10), 785–794.

Fakruddin, M., Hossain, Z., Afroz, H., 2012. Prospects and applications of nanobiotechnology: a medical perspective. *J Nanobiotechnol.* 10, 31.

Fang, L., Wang, H., Zhou, L., Yu, D., 2011. FOXO3a reactivation mediates the synergistic cytotoxic effects of rapamycin and cisplatin in oral squamous cell carcinoma cells. Toxicol. *Appl. Pharmacol.* 251 (1), 8–15.

Figueiró Longo, J., Muehlmann, L., Velloso, N., Simioni, A., Lozzi, S., 2012. Effects of photodynamic therapy mediated by liposomal aluminumphthalocyanine chloride on chemically induced tongue tumors. *Chemotherapy* 1, 103.

Formariz, T. P., Urban, M. C. C., Silva Júnior, A., Gremião, M. P. D., Oliveira, A., 2005. Microemulsões e fases líquidas cristalinas como sistemas de liberação de fármacos. *Rev, Brasil. Ciênc. Farm.* 41, 301–313, In Portuguese. [Microemulsions and liquid crystalline phases as drug delivery systems.]

Freitas, Jr., R. A., 2005a. Nanotechnology, nanomedicine and nanosurgery. Int. J. Surg. 3 (4), 243–246. Freitas, Jr., R. A., 2005b. What is nanomedicine? *Nanomedicine* 1 (1), 2–9.

Gao, Y., Ren, F., Ding, B., Sun, N., Liu, X., Ding, X., Gao, S., 2011. A thermo-sensitive PLGA-PEG-PLGA hydrogel for sustained release of docetaxel. *J. Drug. Target.* 19 (7), 516–527.

Gau, V., Wong, D., 2007. Oral fluid nanosensor test (OFNASET) with advanced electrochemical-based molecular analysis Platform. *Ann. NY Acad. Sci.* 1098 (1), 401–410.

Ghasemiyeh, P.; Mohammadi-samani, S. Solid lipid nanoparticles and nanostructured lipid carriers as novel drug delivery systems: Applications, advantages and disadvantages. *Res. Pharm. Sci.* 2018, 13, 288–303.

Gillenwater A, Papadimitrakopoulou V, Richards-Kortum R. Oral premalignancy: new methods of detection and treatment. *Curr Oncol Rep.* 2006 March;8(2):146–54.

Gupta PC, Warnakulasuriya S. Global epidemiology of areca nut usage. *Addiction Biol.* 2002;7:77–83.

Haddad, R., Sonis, S., Posner, M., Wirth, L., Costello, R., Braschayko, P., Allen, A., Mahadevan, A., Flynn, J., Burke, E., Li, Y., Tishler, R. B., 2009. Randomized phase 2 study of concomitant chemoradiotherapy using weekly carboplatin/paclitaxel with or without daily subcutaneous amifostine in patients with locally advanced head and neck cancer. *Cancer* 115 (19), 4514–4523.

Hao, T., Li, Z., Qiao, M., Fan, Q., Zhang, N., Chen, D., 2009. Preparation of docetaxel hydrogels for subcutaneous injection and their release profile *in vitro*. *Chinese Pharm. J.* 24, 15, In Chinese.

Hatziantoniou, S., Demetzos, C., 2006. Qualitative and quantitative one-step analysis of lipids and encapsulated bioactive molecules in liposome preparations by HPTLC/FID (IATROSCAN). *J. Liposome Res.* 16 (4), 321–330.

Hosmer, J. M., Shin, S. H., Nornoo, A., Sheng, H., Lopes, L. B., 2012. Influence of internal structure and composition of liquid crystalline phases on topical delivery of paclitaxel. *J. Pharm. Sci.* 100 (4), 1444–1455.

Huang B, Chen H, Fan M. A postulated role for human papillomavirus (HPV) in the transformation and proliferation of oral squamous cell carcinoma (OSCC). *Med Hypotheses*. 2008; 70(5):1041–3.

Huang, H.; Barua, S.; Sharma, G.; Dey, S. K.; Rege, K. Inorganic nanoparticles for cancer imaging and therapy. *J. Control. Release* 2011, 155, 344–357.

Huang, X. H., El-Sayed, I. H., Qian, W., El-Sayed, M. A., 2006. Cancer cell imaging and photothermal therapy in the near-infrared region by using gold nanorods. *J. Am. Chem. Soc.* 128 (6), 2115–2120.

Huang, X. H., El-Sayed, I. H., Qian, W., El-Sayed, M. A., 2006. Cancer cell imaging and photothermal therapy in the near-infrared region by using gold nanorods. *J. Am. Chem. Soc.* 128 (6), 2115–2120.

Huang, X. H., El-Sayed, I. H., Qian, W., El-Sayed, M. A., 2006. Cancer cell imaging and photothermal therapy in the near-infrared region by using gold nanorods. *J. Am. Chem. Soc.* 128 (6), 2115–2120.

Huang, X., Jain, P. K., El-Sayed, I. H., El-Sayed, M. A., 2007. Gold nanoparticles: interesting optical properties and recent applications in cancer diagnostics and therapy. *Nanomedicine* 2 (5), 681–693.

Hull, L., Farrell, D., Grodzinski, P., 2014. Highlights of recent developments and trends in cancer nanotechnology research—view from NCI Alliance for nanotechnology in cancer. *Biotechnol. Adv.* 32 (4), 666–678.

Jain, R. K., Stylianopoulos, T., 2010. Delivering nanomedicine to solid tumors. *Nat. Rev. Clin. Oncol.* 7, 653–664.

James, W., Hirsch, L., West, J., O'Neal, P., Payne, J., 2007. Application of INAA to the build-up and clearance of gold nanoshells in clinical studies in mice. *J. Radioanal. Nucl. Chem.* 271 (2), 455–459.

Jawahar, N.; Meyyanathan, S. Polymeric nanoparticles for drug delivery and targeting: A comprehensive review. *Int. J. Heal. Allied Sci.* 2012, 1, 217.

Jones DL, Rankin KV. Oral cancer and associated risk factors. In: Cappelli DP, Mobley CC, editors. *Prevention in Clinical Oral Health Care*. St. Louis, MO: Mosby Elsevier; 2008. Pp. 68–77.

Jordan RC, Daley T. Oral squamous cell carcinoma: new insight. *Cancer Dental Association*. 1997;63(7):517–8, 521–5.

Kang, J. H., Asami, Y., Murata, M., Kitazaki, H., Sadanaga, N., Tokunaga, E., Shiotani, S., Okada, S., Maehara, Y., Nidome, T., 2010. Gold nanoparticlebased colorimetric assay for cancer diagnosis. *Biosens. Bioelectron.* 25, 1869–1874.

Kantola S, Parikka M, Jokinen K, Hyrynkangs K, Soini Y, Alho OP, Salo T. Prognostic factors in tongue cancer–relative importance of demographic, clinical and histopathological factors. *Brit J Cancer.* 2000 Sep; 83(5):61.

Kapse-Mistry, S., Govender, T., Srivastava, R., Yergeri, M., 2014. Nanodrug delivery in reversing multidrug resistance in cancer cells. *Fronti. Pharmacol.* 5 (159).

Khan, Z., Bisen, P. S., 2013. Oncoapoptotic signaling and deregulated target genes in cancers: special reference to oral cancer. *Biochim. Biophys. Acta* 1836, 123–145.

Khosa, A.; Reddi, S.; Saha, R. N. Biomedicine & Pharmacotherapy Nanostructured lipid carriers for site-specific drug delivery. *Biomed. Pharmacother.* 2018, 103, 598–613.

Ko YC, Huang YL, Lee CH, Chen MJ, Lin LM, Tsai CC. Betel quid chewing, cigarette smoking and alcohol consumption related to oral cancer in Taiwan. *J Oral Pathol Med.* 1995 Nov 1;24(10):450–3.

Konishi, M., Tabata, Y., Kariya, M., Hosseinkhani, H., Suzuki, A., Fukuhara, K., Mandai, M., Takakura, K., Fujii, S., 2005. *In vivo* anti-tumor effect of dual release of cisplatin and adriamycin from biodegradable gelatin hydrogel. *J Control. Release* 103 (1), 7–19.

Kruijtzer, C. M. F., Beijnen, J. H., Schellens, J. H. M., 2002. Improvement of oral drug treatment by temporary inhibition of drug transporters and/or cytochrome P450 in the gastrointestinal tract and liver: an overview. *Oncologist* 7 (6), 516–530.

Kulkarni, S. A.; Feng, S. S. Effects of particle size and surface modification on cellular uptake and biodistribution of polymeric nanoparticles for drug delivery. *Pharm. Res.* 2013, 30, 2512–2522. 86. Hoshyar, N.; Gray, S.; Han, H.; Bao, G. The effect of nanoparticle size on *in vivo* pharmacokinetics and cellular interaction. *Nanomedicine* 2016, 11, 673–692.

Kumar, A., Ma, H., Zhang, X., Huang, K., Jin, S., Liu, J., Wei, T., Cao, W., Zou, G., Liang, X. J., 2012a. Gold nanoparticles functionalized with therapeutic and targeted peptides for cancer treatment. *Biomaterials* 33, 1180–1189.

Kumar, R., Kulkarni, A., Nagesha, D. K., Sridhar, S., 2012b. *In vitro* evaluation of theranostic polymeric micelles for imaging and drug delivery in cancer. *Theranostics* 2, 714.

Lian, T., Ho, RJ., 2001. Trends and developments in liposome drug delivery systems. *J. Pharm. Sci.* 90 (6), 667–680.

Lida, S., Shimada, J., Sakagami, H., 2013. Cytotoxicity induced by docetaxel in human oral squamous cell carcinoma cell lines. *In vivo* 27, 321–332.

Lin, Y. K., Huang, Z. R., Zhuo, R. Z., Fang, J. Y., 2010. Combination of calcipotriol and methotrexate in nanostructured lipid carriers for topical delivery. *Int. J. Nanomed.* 5, 117.

Liu, D., Gao, Z., Luo, Q., Wu, Z. S., 2010. Conductive three-dimensional ordered nano-gold film: ultrasensitive electrochemical sensing platform for clinical immunoassay. *Talanta* 82, 1175–1180.

Liu, L., Tang, Y., Gao, C., Li, Y., Chen, S., Xiong, T., Li, J., Du, M., Gong, Z., Chen, H., 2014. Characterization and biodistribution *in vivo* of quercetinloaded cationic nanostructured lipid carriers. *Colloids Surf.* 115, 125–131.

Liu, S. L., Zhong, S. S., Ye, D. X., Chen, W. T., Zhang, Z. Y., Deng, J., 2013. Repression of G protein–coupled receptor family C group 5 member A is associated with pathologic differentiation grade of oral squamous cell carcinoma. *J. Oral Pathol. Med.* 42, 761–768.

Liu, S. L., Zhong, S. S., Ye, D. X., Chen, W. T., Zhang, Z. Y., Deng, J., 2013. Repression of G protein–coupled receptor family C group 5 member A is associated with pathologic differentiation grade of oral squamous cell carcinoma. *J. Oral Pathol. Med.* 42, 761–768.

Mahapatro, A., Singh, D. K., 2011. Biodegradable nanoparticles are excellent vehicle for site directed *in-vivo* delivery of drugs and vaccines. *J. Nanobiotechnol.* 9.

Manmode, A. S., Sakarkar, D. M., Mahajan, N. M., 2009. Nanoparticles-tremendous therapeutic potential: a review. *Intl. J. Pharm. Tech. Res.* 1, 1020–1027.

Manohar, S., Ungureanu, C., Van Leeuwen, T. G., 2011. Gold nanorods as molecular contrast agents in photoacoustic imaging: the promises and the caveats. *Contrast Media Mol. Imaging* 6, 389–400.

Marupudi, N. I., Han, J. E., Li, K. W., Renard, V. M., Tyler, B. M., Brem, H., 2007. Paclitaxel: a review of adverse toxicities and novel delivery strategies. *Expert Opin. Drug Saf.* 6 (5), 609–621.

Moghimi, S. M., Hunter, A. C., Murray, J. C., 2005. Nanomedicine: current status and future prospects. *FASEB J.* 19 (3), 311–330.

Moghimi, S. M., Hunter, A. C., Murray, J. C., 2005. Nanomedicine: current status and future prospects. *FASEB J.* 19 (3), 311–330.

Mohanraj, V.J., Chen, Y., 2006. Nanoparticles – a review. *Trop. J. Pharm. Res.* 5 (1), 561–573.

Mousa, S. A., Bharali, D. J., 2011. Nanotechnology-based detection and targeted therapy in cancer: nano-bio paradigms and applications. *Cancers* 3 (3), 2888–2903.

Mubben, R., Singh, A., 2010. Nanotechnology in the field of oral medicine and diagnosis-a review. *Indian Dent. Res. Rev.* 5, 41–43.

Mukherjee, P., Katarya, A., McMaster, N., Gonzalez, M. A., Bhattacharya, R., 2011. Synthesis of silver nanocubes by photoreduction of silver salts in the presence of proteins. *Int. J. Green Nanotechnol. Biomed.* 3 (2), 134–139.

Myers, E. N., Simental, A. A., 2003. Cancer of the oral cavity. In: Myers, E. N., Suen, J. Y., Myers, J. N., Hanna, E. Y. (Eds.), *Cancer of the head and neck*. Saunders, Philadelphia, PA, pp. 279–332.

Nagahara, L., Tao, N., Thundat, T., 2007. *Introduction to nanosensors.* Springer, New York, NY.

Omar, E., 2015. currentCurrent concepts and future non-invasive procedure for diagnosing oral squamous cell carcinoma a systematic review. *Head Face Med.* 11, 6.

Paciotti, G. F., Kingston, D. G. I., Tamarkin, L., 2006. Colloidal gold nanoparticles: a novel nanoparticle platform for developing multifunctional tumortargeted drug delivery vectors. *Drug Dev. Res.* 67 (1), 47–54.

Paciotti, G. F., Kingston, D. G. I., Tamarkin, L., 2006. Colloidal gold nanoparticles: a novel nanoparticle platform for developing multifunctional tumortargeted drug delivery vectors. *Drug Dev. Res.* 67 (1), 47–54.

Paciotti, G. F., Myer, L., Weinreich, D., Goia, D., Pavel, N., McLaughlin, R. E., Tamarkin, L., 2004. Colloidal gold: a novel nanoparticle vector for tumor directed drug delivery. *Drug Deliv.* 11 (3), 169–183.

Park, J. H., Von Maltzahn, G., Ruoslahti, E., Bhatia, S. N., Sailor, M. J., 2008. Micellar hybrid nanoparticles for simultaneous magnetofluorescent imaging and drug delivery. *Angew. Chem. Intl. Ed. Engl.* 47, 7284–7288.

Park, J. W., 2002. Liposome—based drug delivery in breast cancer treatment. *Breast Cancer Res.* 4 (3), 95–99.

Park, J. W., 2002. Liposome—based drug delivery in breast cancer treatment. *Breast Cancer Res.* 4 (3), 95–99.

Park, J. W., Benz, C. C., Martin, F. J., 2004. Future directions of liposome- and immunoliposome based cancer therapeutics. *Semin. Oncol.* 31, 196–205.

Peer, D., Karp, J. M., Hong, S., Farokhzad, O. C., Margalit, R., Langer, R., 2007. Nanocarriers as an emerging platform for cancer therapy. *Nat. Nanotechnol.* 2 (12), 751–760.

Petersen PE. Oral cancer prevention and control–the approach of the World Health Organization. *Oral Oncol.* 2009 May 31;45(4):454–60.

Popovtzer, R., Agrawal, A., Nicholas, A., et al., 2008. Targeted gold nanoparticles enable molecular CT imaging of cancer. *Nano Lett.* 8 (12), 4593–4596.

Praetorius, N. P., Mandal, T. K., 2007. Engineered nanoparticles in cancer therapy. *Recent Pat. Drug Deliv. Formul.* 1 (1), 37–51.

Pridgen, E. M., Langer, R., Farokhzad, O. C., 2007. Biodegradable, polymeric nanoparticle delivery systems for cancer therapy. *Nanomedicine* 2 (5), 669–680.

Reddy, S. R., Dathar, S., 2015. Nanodrug delivery in oral cancer therapy. an emerging avenue to unveil. *J. Med. Radiol. Pathol. Surg.* 1, 17–22.

Ries, L. A. G., Melbert, D., Krapcho, M., Stinchcomb, D., Howlader, N., Horner, M., Mariotto, A., Miller, B., Feuer, E., Altekruse, S., 2008. *SEER cancer statistics review*, 1975–2005. National Cancer Institute, Bethesda, MD.

Rizvi, S. A. A.; Saleh, A. M. Applications of nanoparticle systems in drug delivery technology. *Saudi Pharm. J.* 2018, 26, 64–70.

Sahoo, S. K., Parveen, S., Panda, J. J., 2007. The present and future of nanotechnology in human health care. *Nanomedicine* 3 (1), 20–31.

Salamat-Miller, N., Chittchang, M., Johnston, T. P., 2005. The use of mucoadhesive polymers in buccal drug delivery. *Adv. Drug Deliv. Rev.* 57 (11), 1666–1691.

Saravana, K. R., Vijayalakshmi, R., 2006. Nanotechnology in dentistry. *Indian J. Dent. Res.* 17 (2), 62–65.

Sato, I.; Umemura, M.; Mitsudo, K.; Fukumura, H.; Kim, J. H.; Hoshino, Y.; Nakashima, H.; Kioi, M.; Nakakaji, R.; Sato, M.; *et al.* Simultaneous hyperthermia-chemotherapy with controlled drug delivery using single-drug nanoparticles. *Sci. Rep.* 2016, 6, 1–12.

Scully, C. (Ed.), 2013. *Oral and Maxillofacial Medicine. theThe basis of diagnosis and treatment.* thirdThird ed Churchill Livingstone, Elsevier, New York, NY, pp. 2014–2017.

Scully, C. (Ed.), 2013. *Oral and Maxillofacial Medicine. theThe basis of diagnosis and treatment.* thirdThird ed Churchill Livingstone, Elsevier, New York, NY, pp. 2014–2017.

Scully, C. (Ed.), 2013. *Oral and Maxillofacial Medicine. theThe basis of diagnosis and treatment.* thirdThird ed Churchill Livingstone, Elsevier, New York, NY, pp. 2014–2017.

Seigneuric, R., Markey, L., Nuyten, D. S., Dubernet, C., Evelo, C. T., Finot, E., Garrido, C., 2010. From nanotechnology to nanomedicine: applications to cancer research. *Curr. Mol. Med.* 10 (7), 640–652.

Sha, M. Y., Xu, H., Penn, S. G., Cromer, R., 2007. SERS nanoparticles: a new optical detection modality for cancer diagnosis. *Nanomedicine* (London), 725–734.

Shaffer, C., 2005. Nanomedicine transforms drug delivery. *Drug Discov. Today* 10 (23–24), 1581–1582.

Shah JP, Lydiatt W. Treatment of cancer of the head and neck. CA Cancer *J Clin.* 1995; 45(6):352–68.

Shah, J. P., Lydiatt, W., 1995. Treatment of cancer of the head and neck. *CA Cancer J. Clin.* 45 (6), 352–368.

Shah, J. P., Lydiatt, W., 1995. Treatment of cancer of the head and neck. *CA Cancer J. Clin.* 45 (6), 352–368.

Shetty, N. J., Swati, P., David, K., 2013. Nanorobots: future in dentistry. *Saudi Dental J.* 25 (2), 49–52.

Shim, M. S., Kim, C. S., Ahn, Y. C., Chen, Z., Kwon, Y. J., 2010. Combined multimodal optical imaging and targeted gene silencing using stimulitransforming nanotheragnostics. *J. Am. Chem. Soc.* 132 (24), 8316–8324.

Sim, R. B.; Wallis, R. Surface properties: Immune attack on nanoparticles. *Nat. Nanotechnol.* 2011, 6, 80.

Sindura, C. S., Babu, N. C., Vinod, 2013. Unbounding the future: nanobiotechnology in detection and treatment of oral cancer. *J. Adv. Med. Dent. Sci. Res.* 1 (2), 66–77.

Singh, G.; Lohani, A.; Bhattacharya, S. S. Hydrogel as a novel drug delivery system: A review. *J. Fundam. Pharm. Res.* 2014, 2, 35–48.

Stewart, B. W., Wild, C. P., 2014. *World cancer report 2014*. IARC, Lyon, France.

Stratton, M. R, 2014. Exploring the genome of cancer cells: progress and promise. *Science* 331, 1553–1558.

Su CC, Yang HF, Huang SJ, Lianie B. Distinctive features of oral cancer in Changhua County: high incidence, buccal mucosa preponderance, and a close relation to betel quid chewing habit. *J Formos Med Assoc.* 2007; 106(3):225–33.

Subramani, K.; Ahmed, W. *Nanoparticulate Drug Delivery Systems for Oral Cancer Treatment,* 1st ed.; Elsevier Inc.: Amsterdam, The Netherlands, 2012;

Sukhija, P., Kamath, G., Babshet, M., Srikanth, H., Bajoria, A. A., 2015. Theranostic gold nanoparticles: a novel approach in head and neck cancer. *IJSS Case Rep. Rev.* 2, 36.

Sumer, B., Gao, J., 2008. Theranostic nanomedicine for cancer. *Nanomedicine* 3 (2), 137–140.

Sun, M.; Su, X.; Ding, B.; He, X.; Liu, X.; Yu, A.; Lou, H.; Zhai, G. Advances in nanotechnology-based delivery systems for curcumin. *Nanomedicine* 2012, 7, 1085–1100.

Sung H, Ferlay J, Siegel RL, Laversanne M, Soerjomataram I, Jemal A, Bray F. Global cancer statistics 2020: GLOBOCAN estimates of incidence and mortality worldwide for 36 cancers in 185 countries. *CA Cancer J Clin*. 2021 Feb 4.

Tang, H. W., Zhang, L. P., Li, S., Zhao, G. J., Qin, Z., Sun, S. Q., 2010. Study on spectroscopic characterization and property of PES/ micro-nano cellulose composite membrane material. *Guang Pu Xue Yu Guang Pu Fen Xi* 30, 630–634, Chinese.

Tang-na, H., Zhen, L., Ming-xi, Q., Qing, F., Ning, Z., Da-wei, C., 2009. Preparation of docetaxel hydrogels for subcutaneous injection and their release profile *in vitro*. *Chinese Pharm. J.* 24, 15.

Tang-na, H., Zhen, L., Ming-xi, Q., Qing, F., Ning, Z., Da-wei, C., 2009. Preparation of docetaxel hydrogels for subcutaneous injection and their release profile *in vitro*. *Chinese Pharm. J.* 24, 15.

Tauro, J. R., Gemeinhart, R. A., 2005. Extracellular protease activation of chemotherapeutics from hydrogel matrices: a new paradigm for local chemotherapy. *Mol. Pharm.* 2 (5), 435–438.

Terwogt, J. M. M., Schellens, J. H. M., Huinink, W. W. t. B., Beijnen, J. H., 1999. Clinical pharmacology of anticancer agents in relation to formulations and administration routes. *Cancer Treat. Rev.* 25 (2), 83–102.

Thomas S, Kearsley J. Betel quid and oral cancer: a review. *Eur J Cancer. Part B, Oral Oncol.* 1993;29B:251–5.

Upadhyay, Y., 2013. Current state and future perspectives of nanotechnology in dentistry. *IOSR J. Pharm.* 3 (9), 68–71.

Velloso, N., Muehlmann, L., Longo, J., Silva, J., Zancanela, D., Tedesco, A., Azevedo, R., 2012. Aluminum-phthalocyanine chloride-based photodynamic therapy inhibits PI3K/Akt/Mtor pathway in oral squamous cell carcinoma cells *in vitro*. *Chemotherapy* 1, 2.

Vermorken, J. B., Mesia, R., Rivera, F., Remenar, E., Kawecki, A., Rottey, S., Erfan, J., Zabolotnyy, D., Kienzer, H. R., Cupissol, D., Peyrade, F., Benasso, M., Vynnychenko, I., De Raucourt, D., Bokemeyer, C., Schueler, A., Amellal, N., Hitt, R., 2008. Platinum-based chemotherapy plus cetuximab in head and neck cancer. *N. Engl. J. Med.* 359 (11), 1116–1127.

Vermorken, J. B., Remenar, E., van Herpen, C., Gorlia, T., Mesia, R., Degardin, M., Stewart, J. S., Jelic, S., Betka, J., Preiss, J. H., van den Weyngaert, D., Awada, A., Cupissol, D., Kienzer, H. R., Rey, A., Desaunois, I., Bernier, J., Lefebvre, J. L., 2007a. Cisplatin, fluorouracil, and docetaxel in unresectable head and neck cancer. *N. Engl. J. Med.* 357 (17), 1695–1704.

Vermorken, J. B., Trigo, J., Hitt, R., Koralewski, P., Diaz-Rubio, E., Rolland, F., Knecht, R., Amellal, N., Schueler, A., Baselga, J., 2007b. Open-label, uncontrolled, multicenter phase II study to evaluate the efficacy and toxicity of cetuximab as a single agent in patients with recurrent and/or metastatic squamous cell carcinoma of the head and neck who failed to respond to platinum-based therapy. *J. Clin. Oncol.* 25 (16), 2171–2177.

Vijayakumar, M. R., Muthu, M. S., Singh, S., 2013. Copolymers of poly (lactic acid) and D-α-tocopheryl polyethylene glycol 1000 succinate-based nanomedicines: versatile multifunctional platforms for cancer diagnosis and therapy. *Expert Opin. Drug Deliv.* 10 (4), 529–543.

Virupakshappa, B., 2012. Applications of nanomedicine in oral cancer. *Oral Health Dent. Manag.* 11 (2), 62–68.

Vogell, S., 2013. Chairside salivary diagnostics for oral diseases. *RDH*, 62–70.

Von Maltzahn, G., Park, J. H., Agrawal, A., Bandaru, N. K., Das, S. K., Sailor, M. J., Bhatia, S. N., 2009. Computationally guided photothermal tumor therapy using long-circulating gold nanorod antennas. *Cancer Res*. 69, 3892–3900.

Wang, J., Dai, Y., Huang, Y., Chen, X., Wang, H., Hong, Y., Xia, J., Cheng, B., 2013. All-trans retinoic acid restores gap junctional intercellular communication between oral cancer cells with upregulation of Cx32 and Cx43 expressions *in vitro*. *Med. Oral Patol. Oral Cir. Bucal* 18, e569.

Warnakulasuriya S, Trivedy C, Peters TJ. Areca nut use: an independent risk factor for oral cancer. *BMJ.* 2002 Apr 6;324(7341):799–800.

Wei, F., Wong, D., 2011. Point-of-care platforms for salivary diagnoostics. *Chin. J. Dent. Res.* 15, 7–15.

Yamada, T., Iwasaki, Y., Tada, H., Iwabuki, H., Chuah, M. K., VandenDriessche, T., Fukuda, H., Kondo, A., Ueda, M., Seno, M., Tanizawa, K., Kuroda, S., 2003. *Nat. Biotechnol.* 8, 885–890.

Yu, D., Wang, A., Huang, H., Chen, Y., 2008b. PEG-PBLG nanoparticle-mediated HSV-TK/GCV gene therapy for oral squamous cell carcinoma. *Nanomedicine* (London) 3 (6), 813–821.

Yu, T., Wood, R. E., Tenenbaum H. C., 2008a. Delays in diagnosis of head and neck cancers. *J. Can. Dent. Assoc*. 74 (1), 61.

Zeng, N., Hu, Q., Liu, Z., Gao, X., Hu, R., Song, Q., Gu, G., Xia, H., Yao, L., Pang, Z., Jiang, X., Chen, J., Fang, L., 2012. Preparation and characterization of paclitaxel-loaded DSPE-PEG-liquid crystalline nanoparticles (LCNPs) for improved bioavailability. *Int. J. Pharm*. 424 (1–2), 58–66.

Zentner, G. M., Rathi, R., Shih, C., McRea, J. C., Seo, M.-H., Oh, H., Rhee, B., Mestecky, J., Moldoveanu, Z., Morgan, M., 2001. Biodegradable block copolymers for delivery of proteins and water-insoluble drugs. *J. Control. Release* 72 (1), 203–215.

Zentner, G. M., Rathi, R., Shih, C., McRea, J. C., Seo, M.-H., Oh, H., Rhee, B., Mestecky, J., Moldoveanu, Z., Morgan, M., 2001. Biodegradable block copolymers for delivery of proteins and water-insoluble drugs. *J. Control. Release* 72 (1), 203–215.

Zlotogorski, A., Dayan, A., Dayan, D., Chaushu, G., Salo, T., Vered, M., 2013. Nutraceuticals as new treatment approaches for oral cancer–I: curcumin. *Oral Oncol.* 49, 187–191.

In: Oral Squamous Cell Carcinoma
Editor: Matthew Rabin
ISBN: 978-1-53619-895-9

Chapter 5

BIOMARKERS: A POWERFUL ARMOR FOR DIAGNOSIS OF ORAL SQUAMOUS CELL CARCINOMA

Jerin Jose* and Diana Daniel
Department of oral and maxillofacial surgery,
The Oxford Dental College, Bangalore, Karnataka, India

ABSTRACT

According to global cancer statistics 2018 (GLOBOCAN 2018), cancer is the second leading cause of death globally. Estimated 18.1 million new cancer cases and 9.6 million cancer deaths. It is most common in India, accounting for 120000 with 90% of oral squamous cell carcinoma (OSCC). The incidence and mortality rate of cancer has shown a sharp increase over the last two decades. Most oral cancers are not diagnosed at an early stage even though they are easily accessible under direct visual examination. Mortality rates remain unchanged despite vast advances in the field of oncology. Therefore, more intense efforts are required to fight against life-threatening diseases and to reduce morbidity and mortality rates.

* Corresponding Author's E-mail: jessicajose19@gmail.com.

Biomarkers are powerful diagnostic tools that can be measured in bodily fluids such as blood, serum, plasma, and body secretions such as saliva. They release certain biochemical substances that are expressed in large quantities at the cell surface by malignant cells. The anatomical proximity of salivary biomarkers to oral cancer makes it the most accurate and specific diagnostic tool and it is a non-invasive alternative to serum testing. More than 100 salivary biomarkers have already been identified, including cytokines (IL-8, IL-1β, and TNF-a), P53, transferrin, DUSP, MMP, and LDH.

In recent years due to the revolution in molecular biology, the development of valid biomarkers has been a breakthrough in the field of cancer research and care. Substantial progress has been made in the development and clinical application of biomarkers and matched targeted therapies. The recent emergence of highly selective technologies has provided global information to observe genetic and proteomic alterations and to facilitate the discovery of new biomarkers with improved sensitivity and specificity. The use of biomarker-based diagnostics for cancer includes non-invasive screening for early-stage disease, detection and localization, risk assessment, disease stratification and prognosis, response to therapy and, for those in remission, screening for disease recurrence. The current chapter aims to elaborate on the importance of biomarkers as an early diagnostic tool in detecting oral squamous cell carcinoma.

Keywords: serum biomarker, oral cancer, salivary biomarker, oral squamous cell carcinoma

INTRODUCTION

OSCC is one of the malignancies with the highest morbidity and mortality rates. To improve survival and reduce the mortality rate diagnosing cancer at the earliest stage is of utmost importance. It is now well accepted that the transition from normal mucosa to invasive squamous cell carcinoma (SCC) is a complex and multistep process, with a multifactorial aetiology [1]. The molecular-level changes that occur in carcinogenesis are: (i) cancer cell proliferation without external stimuli, (ii) insensitivity to inhibitory growth signals, (iii) evasion of apoptosis or cell death mechanisms and/or activation of anti-apoptotic genes, (iv) unlimited replicative potential, (v) sustained angiogenesis, (vi) invasion and metastasis ability, (vii) genomic instability, and (viii) protooncogene mutations caused by defects in DNA repair. These genetic and epigenetic changes disturb the homeostatic equilibrium between cell proliferation and cell death [2]. Despite advances in these clinical treatments, the overall survival rates of OSCC remain generally poor at approximately 50-60% [3, 4]. This is mainly due to frequent late diagnosis in up to 50% of the cases showing lymph node metastasis at the time of the initial clinical investigation. Apart from tumour size, the presence of lymph node metastasis is regarded as the single most important predictor of patient outcomes [5, 6, 7]. In the initial clinical staging, the TNM classification is used; however, it appears to be insufficient to accurately predict tumour aggressiveness or to select treatment modalities on an individual basis. Patients with the same TNM stage may have different clinical behaviours, treatment responses, and even different outcomes [8, 9, 10]. Therefore, a more detailed understanding of the molecular events that potentiate growth and dissemination is necessary and can lead to the discovery of novel biomarkers that predict lymph node metastasis, tumour recurrence and overall survival.

What is a Biomarker?

The World Health Organization defines a biomarker as "any substance, structure or process that can be measured in the body or its products and influence or predict the incidence of outcome or disease" [11]. Biomarkers are elaborated by tumor cells either because of the cause or effect of malignant process [12]. These markers are released into circulation such as blood, other body fluids, or tissues after being synthesized by the tumor or expressed in large quantities at the cell surface by malignant cells. They can be used for estimating disease risk, screening for occult primary cancers, distinguishing benign from malignant findings, determining prognosis, acting as predictors/screening, and monitoring disease status. In recent years due to the revolution in molecular biology, the development of valid biomarkers has been a major breakthrough in the field of cancer research and care. Biomarkers can be derived from one, or a combination, of the following body fluids blood, serum, plasma, and body secretions (sputum, saliva), or excretions (stool, urine). Body fluid samples for biomarker investigation can be obtained by non-invasive, minimally invasive or invasive methods such as biopsied tissues [6].

Biomarkers in OSCC

Biomarkers are broadly classified as genomic, proteomic, or metabolomic. [Figure 1]. Methods of Assessment of Biomarkers have been documented and currently practised methods are as follows: Autofluorescence, Western blotting, Enzyme-linked immunosorbent assay (ELISA), Immunohistochemistry (IHC), 2D gel electrophoresis (2DGE) or 2D liquid chromatography (2DLC). Table 1 shows the biomarker type and detection method used. [Table 1] The study of biomarkers involves epigenetics, proteomics, RNA, and microRNA (miRNA)

Epigenetics

Refers to any heritable modification in gene expression without alteration of the DNA sequence or changes in the genetic code. Heritable modification of DNA occurs through several pathways including alterations in DNA methylation and histone modification. Changes in epigenetic modifications including in DNA methylation and histone modification which are responsible for aberrant gene expression have been proposed as potentially important mechanisms of carcinogenesis [22]. The genes associated with hypermethylation in OSCC include cell-cycle control (p16, p15), apoptosis (p14, death-associated protein kinase [DAPK], p73 and Ras association family [RASSF] 1A), Wnt signalling (APC, WIF1 and RUNX3), cell-cell adhesion (E-cadherin) and DNA-repair (MGMT and hMLH1) genes [23, 24].

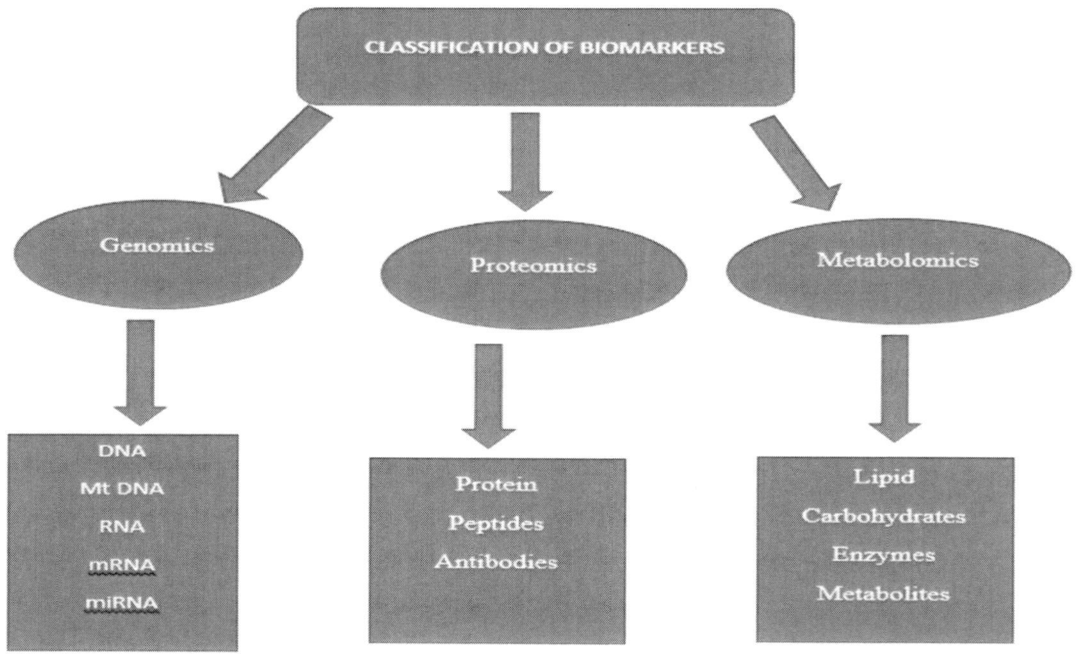
CLASSIFICATION OF BIOMARKERS
Genomics
Proteomics
Metabolomics
DNA
Mt DNA
RNA
mRNA
miRNA
Protein
Peptides
Antibodies
Lipid
Carbohydrates
Enzymes
Metabolites

Figure 1.

Table 1. Demonstrate the biomarker type and detection method

Sl: no	Biomarker category	Serum biomarker	Biomarker type	Detection method
I.	GENOMICS	Mir-483-5p	Rna	Microarray Analysis And (Rt)-Pcr
		Micrornas (Mirnas)Mir-16, Let-7b, Mir-338-3p, Mir-223, And Mir- 29a ., Mir-223 Yielded An Auc Of 0.81 (95% Ci: 0.69–0.92) With 60.0% Specificity And 96.2% Sensitivity, Mir-16 Yielded An Auc Of 0.84 (95% Ci: 0.73–0.94)With 93.3% Specificity And 61.5% Sensitivity, And Let-7b Yielded An Auc Of 0.82 (95% Ci: 0.71–0.93) With 80.0% Specificity And 80.8% Sensitivity.	Rna	Quantitative PCR
I.	GENOMICS	CIRCULATING MICRORNA-21	RNA	QUANTITATIVE REAL TIME RT-PCR
I.	GENOMICS	P53	Gene.	
I.	GENOMICS	C-Erbb-2	Oncogene	Enzyme-Linked Immunosorbent Assay (Elisa)
II.	PROTEOMICS	Cyfra 21-1	Protein	Electrochemiluminescent Immunoassay (Eclia) And Ck19 Messenger Rna (Mrna) Expression In Tissue By Florescent Quantitative Rtpcr
II.	PROTEOMICS	Ceruloplasmin	Glycoprotein	Erba Chem 5 Plus
		Epidermal Growth Factor Receptor (Egfr)	Glycoprotein	Enzyme-Linked Immunosorbent Assay
II.	PROTEOMICS	Sialic Acid	Glycoproteins	Diphenylamine Method
II.	PROTEOMICS	Label-Free Serum Proteomics	Protein	Quantitative Proteomic Analysis (Hdms
II.	PROTEOMICS	Galectin (Gal)-1 And Galectin (Gal)-3	Proteins	Quantitative Real-Time Pcr
II.	PROTEOMICS	Survivin, Carcinoembryonic Antigen (Cea) And Erbb2	Proteins	Usingenzyme-Linked Immunosorbent Assay

Sl: no	Biomarker category	Serum biomarker	Biomarker type	Detection method
II.	PROTEOMICS	Leucine-Rich A2-Glycoprotein (Lrg), Alpha-1-B-Glycoprotein (Abg), Clusterin (Clu), Pro2044, Haptoglobin (Hap), Complement C3c (C3), Proapolipoprotein A1 (Proapo-A1), And Retinol-Binding Protein 4 Precursor (Rbp4)	Proteins	Two-Dimensional Gel Electrophoresis (2-De) And Silver Staining
II.	PROTEOMICS	Growth Differentiation Factor 15 (Gdf15)	Protein	Enzyme-Linked Immunosorbent Assay
II.	PROTEOMICS			
II.	PROTEOMICS	Major Histocompatibility Complex Class I–Related Chain A (Mica)	Protein	Enzyme-Linked Immunoabsorbent Assay
II.	PROTEOMICS	Serum Adenosine Deaminase (Ada)	Protein	Calorimetric Method Of Galanti And Guisti
II.	PROTEOMICS	Albumin	Protein	Electron Paramagnetic Resonance Spectroscopy
II.	PROTEOMICS	Serum N-Glycomes And Anti-Carbohydrate Antibodies	Antibodies	Maldi-Tof-Mass Spectrometry
II.	PROTEOMICS	N-Glycomes And Anti-Carbohydrate Antibodies	Protein And Antibody	Maldi-Tof-Mass Spectrometry
II.	PROTEOMICS	Serum Ferritin, Copper And Zinc	Micronutrients	Immunoenzymatic Kits, Colorimetric Test
II.	PROTEOMICS	Il-6 And/Or Il-8	Glycoprotein	Quantitative Realtime Polymerase Chain Reaction Analysis
III.	METABOLITIES	Fucose	Sugar	Uv-Visible Spectrophotometry Based On The Method As Adopted By Winzler Using Cysteine Reagent
III.	METABOLITIES	Anti–Mmp-7 Antibodies	Proteolytic Enzymes	Real-Time Polymerase Chain Reaction And Western Blot
III.	METABOLITIES	Lactate Dehydrogenase	Enzyme	Autoanalyzer For Spectrometry
III.	METABOLITIES	Serum Il-17f Combined With Vegf	Inflammatory Cytokine	Qrt–Pcr

Table 1. (Continued)

Sl: no	Biomarker category	Serum biomarker	Biomarker type	Detection method
III.	METABOLITIES			
III.	METABOLITIES	Chemerin And Mmp-9	Pro-Angiogenic Factors	Enzyme-Linked Immunosorbent Assays
III.	METABOLITIES	Cxcl12, Cxcr4	Chemokines	Elisa
III.	METABOLITIES	Total Sialic Acid	Monosaccharides	
III.	METABOLITIES	Circulating Immune Complexes, (Copper, Iron And Selenium)	Trace Elements	Oxalyl Dihydrazide Method, Colorimetric DipyridylMethod And The Differential Pulse Cathodic Stripping Voltametry
III.	METABOLITIES	Lipid Bound Sialic Acid	Monosaccharides	Spectrophotometry
III.	METABOLITIES	Metabolomics	Molecules	Nuclear Magnetic Resonance (Nmr) pectroscopy
III.	METABOLITIES	Gdf 15	Growth Factor	Enzyme-Linked Immunosorbent Assay
III.	METABOLITIES	Serum Fucose	Monosaccharides	Cysteine Reagent
III.	METABOLITIES	Serum Levels Of Copper, Iron And Circulating Immune Complexes(Cics)	Molecules	Colorimetric And SpectrophotometricMethods
IV.	GENOMIC &PROTEOMIC	Long Non-Coding Rnas (Lncrnas-Ac007271.3, Ac007182.6, Loc283481, And Rp11-893f2.9), Tumor-Specific Growth Factor(Tsgf), And Squamous Cell Carcinoma Antigen (Scca)	Lncrna Is Rna Scca & Tsgf IsProtein	Lncrna By Microarray Analysis & Real-TimeQuantitative Pcr. Scca & Tsgf By Elisa,

p16INK4a Expression in OSCC

Cell-cycle regulation is crucial in tumorigenesis. This control in eukaryotic cells involves the sequential activation of cyclins, cyclin-dependent kinases (CDKs), and two great CDK inhibitors (CDK-Is): the INK4 family, which comprises inhibitors p16, p15, p18, and p19, and the Cip/Kip family, comprised of p27, p57, and p21Waf1/CIP1. These CDKIs block cell-cycle transition from the G1 phase to the S phase. The inactivation of p16INK4a and p21Waf1/CIP1 has been widely associated with oral cancer and precancer. Sailasree et al. found a relationship between the hypermethylation pattern and increased tumour recurrence; this pattern also acts as an independent predictor agent of poor prognosis [16].

Proteomics

Several tumour-associated proteins, such as stratifin, stathmin, heat shock protein 27, and superoxide dismutase 2 (SOD2). Salivary proteomics in the detection of OSCC includes cytokines (IL-6, IL-8, and IL-β1), cytokeratin 19 fragments (Cyfra21–1), cancer antigen 125 (CA-125):, tissue polypeptide antigen (TPS), and anti-p53 antibodies are frequently found to be altered in HNSCC

Tumour development and progression are complex processes involving oncogenes, tumour suppressor genes, and tumour microenvironment, through their contact with malignant cells, surrounding stromal cells (fibroblasts, endothelial cells, and inflammatory cells), and the extracellular matrix (ECM), formed by structural proteins (such as collagen and elastin), specialized proteins (such as fibrillin, fibronectin, and laminin), and proteoglycans. Several proteases are responsible for remodelling the ECM that enable dissemination and metastasis of tumour cells, such as serine proteases, cysteine cathepsins, and MMPs [26]. There is a group of specific and strong MMPs called endogenous tissue inhibitors of metalloproteinases (TIMPs), although the expression of MMPs has been largely described in almost all tumours of the body, the expression of TIMPs has been studied to a lesser degree and even less in the case of OSCCs.

RNA and MicroRNA

RNA and miRNA are also being used for the identification of altered gene expression in cancer. Nucleic acids can be isolated and detected in blood, urine, cerebrospinal fluid, and saliva using reverse transcription-10 chain reaction detection. This method can be used as a biomarker for cancer diagnosis. Differentially expressed mRNA transcripts between cancer and normal patients' salivary samples could be identified as potential biomarkers for cancer detection, such as DUSPI, H3F3A, OA21, S100P-SAT, IC8, and ILIB. Aberrantly expressed mRNA transcripts exhibited at least a 3.5-fold increase in cancer patients, and the combination of the biomarker panel yielded a sensitivity and specificity of 90% in distinguishing oral HNSCC from the control [16].

IL-8 and IL-1B

IL-8 has been linked to cancer due to its angiogenic properties and its ability to induce cell proliferation and promote DNA damage through the inhibition of DNA repair. It has been proposed that higher levels of IL-8 may promote carcinogenesis not only by inducing cell proliferation and DNA damage but also by upregulating gene in the transcription and activity of metalloproteinase-2. Increased collagenase activity results in an enhanced invasion of surrounding healthy tissues by tumour cells, increased angiogenesis, and, therefore, metastasis.

IL-1β is a cytokine protein encoded by the IL-1B gene in humans. This cytokine is produced by activated macrophages and is processed to its active form by caspase 1. IL-1β exerts various biological functions. Besides, regulating inflammatory response, this cytokine plays a significant role in the development of cancer. IL-1β acts as a potent promoter of tumorigenesis by enhancing the action of chemical carcinogens, which results in the proliferation of mutated cells and further accumulation of genetic damage.

DUSP1

It is considered a negative regulator of cellular proliferation and a regulator of cytokine biosynthesis in responses to bacterial lipopolysaccharide [17]. DUSP1 also plays a significant role in immune regulation and mediates the anti-inflammatory response to glucocorticoids [18]. Several studies have also shown that DUSP1 significantly influences metabolic homeostasis and lipid metabolism [30] also has been shown that DUSP1 protects the oral cavity against inflammation of bacterial aetiology. In recent years, there has been increasing evidence regarding the correlation between altered expression of DUSP1 and cancer. DUSP1 has been implicated as a mediator of the tumour suppressor signalling pathway. It has been suggested that DUSP1 can act as a tumour regulator according to cancer type and stage.

S100 Calcium Binding Protein p

S100P is a 95 amino acid member of the S100 family of proteins and plays a role in protein binding and calcium ion binding. S100P expression has been described in many different cancers and is associated with drug resistance, metastasis, and poor clinical outcomes. In OSCC patients, S100P expressions were elevated.

Epidermal Growth Factor Receptor

The epidermal growth factor receptor (EGFR) is a tyrosine kinase receptor that belongs to the Erb B family of cell receptors. This has many downstream signalling targets. When activated, the receptor can signal via multiple pathways such as MAPK, Akt, RK, and JAB/sTAT. These pathways are related to cellular proliferation, apoptosis, invasion, angiogenesis, and metastasis. EGFR is an important step in tumorigenesis and is a useful molecular marker because its elevated expression levels confer poor survival. It is a promising marker and has significant prognostic value in HNSCC.

Ornithine Decarboxylase Antizyme 1

Catalyzes the conversion of ornithine to putrescine. Initially, it binds to and destabilizes ornithine decarboxylase, which is finally degraded. It also inhibits the cellular uptake of polyamines by inactivating the polyamine uptake transporter. OSCC patients have been found to have significant alterations of serum and salivary OAZ1 compared with healthy controls [19].

Clinical Implication of Biomarkers in Detection of OSCC

Biomarkers have gained immense clinical importance because of their wide spectrum in early detection, diagnosis, prevention, and treatment of cancer. Based on their use, biomarkers can be divided into different categories. The first one includes biomarkers for early detection and screening of patients; the second category consists of diagnostic biomarkers used to detect the presence/absence of cancer; the third one includes prognostic biomarkers to assess the survival probabilities of patients or to detect the aggressive phenotype. The fourth category includes predictive biomarkers to predict the effectiveness of drug treatment and the fifth consists of a target that is used to identify the molecular targets of novel therapies and to know which molecular markers are expressed and affected by therapy [20, 21]. There are a handful of cancer biomarkers that are currently recommended for monitoring treatment response among cancer patients with advanced disease [22].

Oral squamous cell carcinoma (OSCC) represents the sixth most common cancer, accounts for 95% of all oral cavity and oropharyngeal cancers worldwide with approximately 300,000 new cases per year [23]. Most OSCCs are not diagnosed at an early stage even though it is easily accessible for direct visual examination. This event underscores the timely and accurate detection by clinicians to reduce its morbidity and mortality rate. Substantial progress has been made from the discovery to the development and clinical application of biomarkers and matched targeted therapies [24]. Biomarker targeted therapy; for example, EGFR targeted therapy for lung cancer, wild type KRAS for colon cancer, ERBB2 for breast cancer, BRAF for melanoma is already in practice as a standard treatment protocol [25]. Some other biomarkers that have been effectively used in the diagnosis and prognosis of different types of cancers are prostate-specific antigen (PSA) for prostate cancer, alpha-fetoprotein for hepatocellular carcinoma, BRCA1 and BRCA2 for breast cancer, and heat shock proteins for gastric and prostate carcinomas, osteosarcomas, and uterine, cervical, and bladder carcinoma [26].

Table 2. Demonstrates sensitivity and specificity of serum biomarkers in detection of OSCC

Sl : no	Lead author	Biomarker	Biomarker type	Detection method	Sensitivity	Specificity
1.	Tao Jiang [29]	Anti–Mmp-7Antibodies	Proteolytic Enzymes	Real-Time Polymerase Chain Reaction And WesternBlot	0.485	0.896
2.	Huanxi Xu [30]	Mir-483-5p	Rna	Microarray Analysis And (Rt)-Pcr	0.853	0.746
3.	Rewa Malhotra [31]	Cyfra 21-1	Protein	Electrochemiluminescent Immunoassay (Eclia) And Ck19 Messenger Rna (Mrna) Expression In Tissue ByFlorescent Quantitative Rtpcr	88	78.2%,
4.	Noha A. Ghallab [28]	Chemerin And Mmp-9	Pro-Angiogenic Factors	Enzyme-Linked Immunosorbent Assays	100	100
5.	Maximilian Moergel [32]	Albumin	Protein	Electron Paramagnetic Resonance Spectroscopy	72%	80%
6.	Sara Ann Maclellan [33]	Micrornas	Rna	Quantitative Pcr	72%	80.0%
7	Cheng-Zhe Yang [34]	Growth Differentiation Factor 15 (Gdf15)	Protein	Enzyme-Linked Immunosorbent Assay	0.75	0.867
8.	Shigehiro Tamaki[35]	Major Histocompatibility Complex Class I–RelatedChain A (Mica)	Protein	Enzyme-Linked Immunoabsorbent Assay	61.50%	51.00%
9.	Stefano Tiziani [36]	Metabolomics	Molecules	Nuclear Magnetic Resonance (Nmr) Spectroscopy	>95%	>95%
10.	Maie A. R. St. John [37]	Il-6 And/Or Il-8	Glycoprotein	Quantitative Realtime Polymerase Chain Reaction Analysis	Il-8 Saliva Protein = 86 Il-6 Serum Protein = 57 Il-8 Saliva Protein = 99	Il-8 Saliva Protein = 97Il-6 Serum Protein = 100 Il-8 Saliva Protein = 90

Table 2. (Continued)

Sl : no	Lead author	Biomarker	Biomarker type	Detection method	Sensitivity	Specificity
11.	Yang Li, [38]	Rna Biomarkers	Rna	Quantitative Polymerase Chain Reaction (Pcr)	Sensitivity (91%)	Specificity (71%)
12.	Chia-Jung Yu [37]	Gbp1		One-Dimensional Gel Electrophoresis In Combination With The Nano Liquid Chromatography Tandem Mass Spectrometry (Gelc Ms/Ms) Approach	Gbp1 = 78.9%	Gbp1 = 54.1%,
13.	Ashish Gupta [38]	Metabolites	Molecules	H Nuclearmagnetic Resonance (1h Nmr) BasedMetabolomics	Glutamine, Propionate, Acetone, And Choline Of Cancer Cases 93.5% Hc Vs. Oscc = 8 93.8% 0.980 90.9% 96.0%	Glutamine, Propionate, Acetone, And CholineOf Cancer Cases 93.5%

Sensitivity and Specificity of Biomarkers

An ideal biomarker should possess the following characterises of accuracy, reliability, safety, reproducibility, low cost. Besides, it should be quantifiable in an accessible biological fluid and clinical sample with consistency across gender and ethnic groups. A biomarker ideally should possess 100% specificity and sensitivity. A receiver operating curve is used to represent the relationship between specificity and sensitivity. This curve helps to evaluate the efficacy of tumour markers at various cutoff points [27]. The area under the curve (AUC) is taken into consideration. One of the best serum biomarkers (PSA) is used for the detection of prostate cancer. PSA has been found to have high sensitivity (more than 90%) but low specificity (25%). Another serum biomarker, like CA 15.3 for breast cancer, has only 23% sensitivity and 69% specificity, which is used in monitoring therapy for the recurrence of breast cancer.

Serum biomarkers can be useful in the diagnosis of oral squamous cell carcinoma. Despite the increasing number of researches done on biomarkers for OSCC, there is no clear evidence regarding which assays constitute the most accurate type of biomarker (i.e., proteins, nucleic acids, or metabolites), which possess the best diagnostic value, or which is best detection method to use. A review of 14 serum biomarkers for OSCC detection with sensitivity and specificity is summarised in Table 2 [Table 2] Biomarker chemerin and MMP-9 shows excellent sensitivity and specificity which is 100% each. Chemerin also called tazarotene -induced gene 2, is a novel member of adipokines. They are found as the natural ligand of the previously orphan receptor ChemR23. In plasma, they circulate as prochemerin (inactive precursor) which is activated by extracellular proteases. Chemerin stimulate intracellular signal path such as p38 causing the regulation and induction of proinflammatory cytokines such as interleukin-1β and tumour necrosis factor-alpha. MMP-9 is a family of zinc-dependent endopeptidases. Studies have reported that MMP-9 polymorphism is associated with an increased risk for developing oral cancer [28]. Anti MMP antibodies are the ones with the least sensitivity (48.5%).

The detection of OSCC through noninvasive techniques as exfoliative cytology is an alternative option to serum testing. It is a viable methodology for finding and forecasting the expectation of different illnesses. The anatomical proximity of the saliva to oral cancer makes it the most accurate and specific diagnostic tool. In–addition, it can be obtained non-invasively, and inexpensive compared with invasive tissue biopsies. Saliva has been found to reflect the diseased or physiological state of the human body, and hence could be utilized for diagnostic purpose. More than 100 salivary biomarkers have already been identified, including cytokines (IL-8, IL-1β, TNF-a), P53, transferrin, DUSP, MMP, LDH, and many more. Even though there is an exponential increase in the discovery of these several promising diagnostic biomarkers over the last two decades only a few of these biomarkers have been translated into clinical practice especially in the field of carcinogenesis. Several barriers such as poor quality control and lack of samples for validating and testing procedures during the development results in less efficient diagnostics and unpredictability in the clinical outcome of cancer. Although there is an extensive number of examinations on salivary biomarkers and OSCC, a precise survey is important to figure out which of the various accumulations of detailed biomarkers displays satisfactory indicative test exactness. A review of 32 salivary biomarkers with sensitivity and specificity are summarised in Table 3 [Table 3]. MASPIN, CYCD1 showed 100% sensitivity and specificity with ELISA as the detection method. This is because of following a proper standardization procedure for saliva sample collection, processing, and storage. Followed by MMP1 with sensitivity and specificity of 93.5% and 97.8% respectively, when detected by the RT- qPCR method. DUSP1 showed the least sensitivity of 0.14 when PCR AND ELISA were used as the detection method. Lactate dehydrogenase showed the least specificity values when detected by ELISA, Kinetic spectrophotometry due to a lack of standardization for the saliva sample collection, processing and storage

Shen Hu et al. [44]. Demonstrated a subtractive proteomics approach to profile proteins in pooled saliva samples from 16 OSCC and 16 healthy subjects with very well matched in terms of gender, ethnicity, and age to minimize potential bias. The study concluded that the target proteins with soluble CD44, cytokeratin 19 fragment Cyfra21-1, tissue polypeptide showed a sensitivity of 90% and specificity of 83%.

T Shpitzer et al. [19]. Showed that the sensitivity values of the eight analysed markers were in the range of 58–100%whereas the specificity values were in the range of 42–100%. The sensitivity and specificity values were especially high for the CycD1 and Maspin markers, 100% for each value of each marker. These were also quite high for the carbonyls 90% and 80%, respectively, and for the MMP-9 100% and 79%, respectively. This suggests that all eight biomarkers analysed in OSCC patients are highly desirable and beneficial if salivary tumour marker analysis could be performed on a routine basis. Furthermore, salivary biomarkers being noninvasive, and an effective alternative to serum testing, helps in detecting the OSCC at the earliest stage which will then further reduce the morbidity and mortality rate.

Table 3. Showing studies with sensitivity and specificity of salivary biomarkers in OSCC detection

Sl: no	Salivary marker	Detection method	Author name and year	Sensitivity	Specificity
1.	Lactate dehydrogenase	(ELISA, LDH activity by kinetic spectrophotometry	T Shpitzer, 2009 [40]	79	42
2.	MMP1	RT-qPCR	Benjamin Lallemant, 2009 [41]	93.5	97.8
		Multiplex LC-MRM-MS	Jau-Song Yu, 2016 [42]	69.5	95
3.	SPARC	RT-qPCR	Benjamin Lallemant, 2009[41]	71.7	93.5
		Multiplex LC-MRM-MS	Jau-Song Yu, 2016	56.5	86.4
4.	KNG1	BCA	Yi -Ting Chen, 2017 [43]	0.738	0.793
		Protein Assay Kit, Multiplex LC-MRM-MS	Jau-Song Yu, 2016 [42]	84	75.4
5.	CD44	ELISA assay	Elizabeth J. Franzmann, 2007 [46]	62% to 70%	75 to 88%
5.	CD44	Sandwich ELISA,assay Multiplex LC-MRM-MS Reversed-phase liquid chromatography, LC-tandem mass spectrometry, 2D Quant kit, ELISA	Lutécia H. Mateus Pereira, 2017 [47] Jau-Song Yu, 2016 [42] Shen Hu1, 2008 [44] Shen Hu1, 2008 [44]	80.7 76.3 90 90	48.7 57 83.8 83
6.	DUSP1	RiboAmp RNA Amplification kit, Human Genome,Quantitative Polymerase Chain Reaction, U133A Array	Yang Li, 2004 [46]	59	65
		PCR and ELISA	Ole Brinkmann, 2011 [48]	0.14	0.98

Table 3. (Continued)

Sl: no	Salivary marker	Detection method	Author name and year	Sensitivity	Specificity
		(qPCR)	David Elashoff, 2013	0.6	0.56
7.	H3F3A	RiboAmp RNA Amplification kit,			
		Human Genome,Quantitative Polymerase Chain Reaction U133A Array	Yang Li, 2004 [46]	53	81
		(qPCR)	David Elashoff, 2013 [49]	0.61	0.56
8.	IL1B	RiboAmp RNA Amplification kit,			
		Human Genome,Quantitative Polymerase Chain Reaction	Yang Li, 2004 [46]	63	72
		U133A Array			
9.	IL-8	PCR and ELISA	Ole Brinkmann, 2011 [48]	0.23	0.94
	IL-8	(qPCR)	David Elashoff, 2013 [49]	0.65	0.6
	IL-8	PCR and ELISA	Ole Brinkmann, 2011 [48]	0.6	0.78
	IL-8	(qPCR)	David Elashoff, 2013	0.68	0.64
	IL-8	ELISA	Rajkumar. K, 2014 [50]	85%	93%
10.	S100P	RiboAmp RNA Amplification kit,			
		Human Genome,Quantitative Polymerase Chain Reaction	Yang Li, 2004 [46]	72	63
		U133A Array			
		PCR and ELISA	Ole Brinkmann, 2011 [48]	0.54	0.88
		(qPCR)	David Elashoff, 2013	0.6	0.56

Sl: no	Salivary marker	Detection method	Author name and year	Sensitivity	Specificity
11.	SAT	RiboAmp RNA Amplification kit,			
		Human Genome,Quantitative Polymerase Chain Reaction	Yang Li, 2004 [46]	81	56
		U133A Array			
		PCR and ELISA	Ole Brinkmann, 2011 [48]	0.54	0.82
		(qPCR)	David Elashoff, 2013 [49]	0.66	0.63
12.	MMP-9	ELISA, LDH activity by kinetic spectrophotometry	T Shpitzer, 2009 [40]	100	79
		ELISA	Andre Peisker, 2017 [51]	100	79
		Multiplex LC-MRM-MS	Jau-Song Yu [42]	75.6	
13.	Lactic acid	Mass spectrometry	Qihui Wang, 2014 [52]	100	73.3
		Ultraperformance liquid chromatography	Jie Wei, 2010 [53]	73	70.6
14.	OAZ1	Riboamp – RNA amplification, QPCR Q-PCR	Yang Li, 2004 [46] David Elashoff, 2013 [49]	100 62	38 58
15.	HPV 16	Q PCR	AliceY Chuang, 2008 [55]	50	100
16. **17.** **18.** **19.**	FNI IL1RN KRT13 KRT4	Rt- QPCR Rt- QPCR Rt- QPCR Rt- QPCR	Benjamin Lallemant, 2009 [41] Benjamin Lallemant, 2009 [41] Benjamin Lallemant, 2009 [41]	58.7 93.5 75 89.4	76.1 95.7 95.5 91.3
20.	MAL	Rt- QPCR	Benjamin Lallemant, 2009 [41]	95.7	91.3
21.	PLAU	Rt- QPCR	Benjamin Lallemant, 2009 [41]	80.5	89.1
22.	TGM3	Rt- QPCR	Benjamin Lallemant, 2009 [41]	84.8	91.8
23.	CARBONYL	ELISA	T Shpitzer, 2009 [40]	90	80
24.	OGG1	ELISA	T Shpitzer, 2009 [40]	77	75

Table 3. (Continued)

Sl: no	Salivary marker	Detection Method	Author name and year	Sensitivity	Specificity
25.	PHOSPHO-SRC	ELISA	T Shpitzer, 2009 [40]	77	75
26.	KI67	ELISA	T Shpitzer, 2009 [40]	58	67
27.	MASPIN	ELISA	T Shpitzer, 2009 [40]	100	100
28.	CYCD1	ELISA	T Shpitzer, 2009 [40]	100	100
29.	L-leucine	Electrospray ionization	Qihui Wang, 2014 [52]	84.6	81.7
		fluorescence spectroscopic		88.9	94
30.	Ethidium bromide	Multiplex LC-MRM-MS	Manoharan Yuvaraj, 2014 [54]	80.2	68.3
				76.3	60.8
31.	ANXA2		Jau-Song Yu, 2016 [42]	77.1	52.3
	CA2	Multiplex LC-MRM-MS		36.6	77.9
	CRNN		Jau-Song Yu, 2016 [42]	93.1	9.5
	CST3			90.1	47.2
	CSTA			71.8	67.3
	DSG3			61.8	81.9
	FLNA			60.3	73.4
	FSCN1			84.0	67.3
	GANAB			67.9	39.7
	GSTP1				72.4
	IGFBP			68.7	
	ISG15			52.7	95.0, 76.9
	LDHA			93.1	69.3
	MMP1,			69.5.0, 62.6	86.4
	MMP3			69.5	
	S100A9			56.5	
	STAT1				

Sl: no	Salivary marker	Detection Method	Author name and year	Sensitivity	Specificity
32.	A1AG1	BCA protein assaykit	Yi-Ting Chen, 2017 [43]	0.869	0.793
	AACT			0.639	0.759
	ANGT			82.41	0.672
	ANT3			0.672	0.776
	APOB			0.738	0.776
	APOH			0.803	0.845
	C1			0.639	0.914
	CFAH		Yi-Ting Chen, 2017 [43]	0.869	0.845
	CRP	BCA protein assaykit		0.541	0.931
	FA12			0.787	0.741
	FETUA			0.705	0.897
	FIBB			0.721	0.81
	FINC			0.787	0.81
	HEMO			0.754	0.81
	HEP2			0.803	0.914
	HPT			0.721	0.741
	HRG			0.689	0.897
	ITIH1			0.754	0.828
	PLMN			0.738	0.793
	SAA4			0.639	0.793
	SAMP			0.770	0.897
	VTNC			0.721	0.914

Brinkmann, O. et al. [48]. Showed that three proteomes (IL1B, IL8, M2BP) and Four transcriptomes (IL8, IL1B, SAT1, S100P) were significantly elevated ($p < 0.05$) in OSCC patients. The sensitivity/ specificity for OSCC total was 0.89/0.78, for T1-T2 0.67/0.96, and for T3-T4 0.82/0.84. These salivary biomarkers are highly promising and recommended for OSCC detection.

Rajkumar et al. [50]. Showed that the sensitivity and specificity of IL8 are 85% and 93% respectively. The study supports the utility of salivary IL-8 as a marker for routine diagnosis of OSCC and it also suggests that salivary IL-8 can be used as a screening marker of oral cancers.

Andre Peisker et al. [51]. Showed that the sensitivity value of MMP-9 was 100% whereas the specificity value was 26.7%. The data indicate that the elevation of salivary levels of MMP-9 may be a useful adjunctive diagnostic tool for detection of OSCC. However, the specificity values were much reduced due to lack of the standardization and methods used for the detection of the biomarker

Qihui Wang et al. [52]. Showed the sensitivity of 84.6% and specificity of 81.7%. The possibility of salivary metabolite biomarkers for OSCC diagnosis is successfully demonstrated in this study as it is non-invasive, simple, reliable, and also provides lower detection limits and excellent precision and a simple clinical tool for the early diagnosis of OSCC.

Challenges in Developing a Reliable Biomarker for Detection of OSCC

The reliable cancer biomarker should create an absolute true positivity and should produce valid and reliable results of the malignancy type without any confounding factors between malignant and nonmalignant tissue. The cancer tissue undergoes mutational changes and leads to the emergence of a subpopulation of cancer cells known as clones. During cancer progression due to genetic and epigenetic changes of these clonal cells they expand and form new clones termed “clonal diversity resulting in a heterogeneous population of cells this would challenge the development of biomarkers further complicate cancer detection strategies [56].

Studies conducted on genetic assays suggests genes are overexpressed in malignant tissues compared with benign tissues or precursor lesions, and no transcripts or proteins have been identified to be uniquely elevated in cancer. Most of the biomarkers belong to pathways in cell proliferation, cell differentiation, apoptosis, angiogenesis, cell death, and inflammation. Thus, biomarkers expressed in the nucleus or cytoplasm is not accessible, and attention is therefore paid to the cell surface or secreted proteins. Furthermore, transcript proteins are expressed in relatively increased levels, and therefore fail as candidate biomarkers because of low-level expression.

Cancer tissues are complex tissues composed of malignant cells, nonmalignant cells, and inflammatory cells in a tumour microenvironment. It is most likely that the host immune response to the malignancy and the interactions of malignant cells to surrounding stroma are not captured by biomarkers. Thus, focusing on genetic mutations and structural alterations in malignant cells will yield limited predicting behaviour.

Furthermore, many biomarkers fail to validate as reliable ones because of clonal diversity, genomic instability, sample tissue selection, ethnicity, anatomic subsites, detection method, host response and the lack of unique expression of the genomic or proteomic component in cancer tissue.

CONCLUSION

With the current understanding of the pathways associated with tumour initiation and progression, the identification of the potential biomarkers and their utilization for diagnosis in clinical practice Firstly enables to design of a treatment plan for oral cancer. Secondly, it enables to development of biomarkers targeting oral cancer drug therapy. However, further research should be done focussing on identifying and categorizing oral cancer biomarkers in the following areas: Screening, differential diagnosis, recurrence predictor, prognosis, therapeutic, and metastases. This would further aid in determining clinical outcomes and developing dental public health strategies by adhering to the principles and protocols of analytic validity, clinical validity and utility.

REFERENCES

[1] Scully, C., Sudbø, J. & Speight, P. M. (2003). Progress in determining the malignant potential of oral lesions. *Journal of oral pathology & medicine: official publication of the International Association of Oral Pathologists and the American Academy of Oral Pathology*, *32*(5), 251–256. https://doi.org/10.1034/j.1600-0714.2003.00108.x.

[2] Vadas, M., Xia, P., McCaughan, G. & Gamble, J. (2008). The role of sphingosine kinase 1 in cancer: oncogene or non-oncogene addiction?. *Biochimica et biophysica acta*, *1781*(9), 442–447. https://doi.org/10.1016/j.bbalip.2008.06.007.

[3] Seki, S., Fujiwara, M., Matsuura, M., Fujita, S., Ikeda, H., Asahina, I. & Ikeda, T. (2011). Prediction of outcome of patients with oral squamous cell carcinoma using vascular invasion and the strongly positive expression of vascular endothelial growth factors. *Oral oncology*, *47*(7), 588–593. https://doi.org/10.1016/ j.oraloncology.2011.04.013.

[4] Tang, J. Y., Hsi, E., Huang, Y. C., Hsu, N. C., Yang, W. C., Chang, H. W., Chai, C. Y. & Chu, P. Y. (2015). Overexpression of autophagy-related 16-like 1 in patients with oral squamous cell carcinoma. *Pathology oncology research: POR*, *21*(2), 301–305. https://doi.org/10.1007/s12253-014-9821-7.

[5] Hsu, Y. P., Hsieh, C. H., Chien, H. T., Lai, C. H., Tsao, C. K., Liao, C. T., Kang, C. J., Wang, H. M., Chang, J. T. & Huang, S. F. (2015). Serum markers of CYFRA 21-1 and C-reactive proteins in oral squamous cell carcinoma. *World journal of surgical oncology*, *13*, 253. https://doi.org/10.1186/s12957-015-0656-9.

[6] Kono, M., Watanabe, M., Abukawa, H., Hasegawa. O., Satomi, T. & Chikazu, D. (2013) Cyclo-oxygenase-2 expression is associated with

vascular endothelial growth factor C expression and lymph node metastasis in oral squamous cell carcinoma. *J Oral Maxillofac Surg*, *71*, 1694-1702. https://doi.org/10.1016/j.joms.2013.04.015.

[7] Sagheb, K., Blatt, S., Rahimi-Nedjat, R. K., Eigenbrodt, S., Al-Nawas, B. & Walter, C. (2017). Cervical metastases behavior of T1-2 squamous cell cancer of the oral mucosa. *Clinical oral investigations*, *21*(3), 931–935. https://doi.org/10.1007/s00784-016-1845-9.

[8] Fu, T. Y., Hsieh, I. C., Cheng, J. T., Tsai, M. H., Hou, Y. Y., Lee, J. H., Liou, H. H., Huang, S. F., Chen, H. C., Yen, L. M., Tseng, H. H. & Ger, L. P. (2016). Association of OCT4, SOX2, and NANOG expression with oral squamous cell carcinoma progression. *Journal of oral pathology & medicine: official publication of the International Association of Oral Pathologists and the American Academy of Oral Pathology*, *45*(2), 89–95. https://doi.org/10.1111/ jop.12335.

[9] Gissi, D. B., Morandi, L., Gabusi, A., Tarsitano, A., Marchetti, C., Cura, F., Palmieri, A., Montebugnoli, L., Asioli, S., Foschini, M. P. & Scapoli, L. (2018). A Noninvasive Test for MicroRNA Expression in Oral Squamous Cell Carcinoma. *International journal of molecular sciences*, *19*(6), 1789. https://doi.org/10.3390/ ijms19061789.

[10] Oliveira-Costa J., Carvalho A. Fiorini de, Silveira G. Gobbi da, Amaya P., Wu Y., Jenny Park K., Gigliola M. Pinilla, Lustberg M., Cavicchioli Buim M., Ferreira E. Napolitano, Kowalski L. Paulo, Chalmers J. J., Soares F. Augusto., et al. (2015). Gene expression patterns through oral squamous cell carcinoma development: PD-L1 expression in primary tumor and circulating tumor cells. *Oncotarget.*, *6*, 20902-20920. Retrieved from https://www.oncotarget.com/ article/3939/.

[11] Goossens, N., Nakagawa, S., Sun, X. & Hoshida, Y. (2015). Cancer biomarker discovery and validation. *Translational cancer research*, *4*(3), 256–269. https://doi.org/10.3978/j.issn.2218-676X.2015.06.04.

[12] Fernández-Olavarría, A., Mosquera-Pérez, R., Díaz-Sánchez, R. M., Serrera-Figallo, M. A., Gutiérrez-Pérez, J. L. & Torres-Lagares, D. (2016). The role of serum biomarkers in the diagnosis and prognosis of oral cancer: A systematic review. *Journal of clinical and*

experimental dentistry, *8*(2), e184–e193. https://doi.org/10.4317/jced.52736.

[13] Hema, K. N., Smitha, T., Sheethal, H. S. & Mirnalini, S. A. (2017). pigenetics in oral squamous cell carcinoma. *Journal of oral and maxillofacial pathology JOMFP*, *21*(2), 252–259. https://doi.org/10.4103/jomfp.JOMFP_150_17.

[14] Shaw R. (2006). The epigenetics of oral cancer. *International journal of oral and maxillofacial surgery*, *35*(2), 101–108. https://doi.org/10.1016/j.ijom.2005.06.014.

[15] Supic, G., Jovic, N., Kozomara, R., Zeljic, K. & Magic, Z. (2011). Interaction between the MTHFR C677T polymorphism and alcohol--impact on oral cancer risk and multiple DNA methylation of tumor-related genes. *Journal of dental research*, *90*(1), 65–70. https://doi.org/10.1177/0022034510385243.

[16] O'Donnell, R., Kupferman, M., Wei, S., et al. (2005). Gene expression signature predicts lymphatic metastasis in squamous cell carcinoma of the oral cavity. *Oncogene*, *24*, 1244–1251 https://doi.org/10.1038/sj.onc.1208285.

[17] Huang, G., Wang, Y., Shi, L. Z., Kanneganti, T. D. & Chi, H. (2011). Signaling by the phosphatase MKP-1 in dendritic cells imprints distinct effector and regulatory T cell fates. *Immunity*, *35*(1), 45–58. https://doi.org/10.1016/j.immuni.2011.05.014.

[18] Hammer, M., Mages, J., Dietrich, H., Schmitz, F., Striebel, F., Murray, P. J., Wagner, H. & Lang, R. (2005 Oct). Control of dual-specificity phosphatase-1 expression in activated macrophages by IL-10. *Eur J Immunol.*, *35*(10), 2991-3001. doi: 10.1002/eji.200526192. PMID: 16184516.

[19] Shpitzer, T., Bahar, G., Feinmesser, R. & Nagler, R. M. (2007). A comprehensive salivary analysis for oral cancer diagnosis. *Journal of Cancer Research and Clinical Oncology*, *133*, 613–617.

[20] Cervino, G., Fiorillo, L., Herford, A. S., Romeo, U., Bianchi, A., Crimi, S., D'Amico, C., De Stefano, R., Troiano, G., Santoro, R., Laino, L., Laino, G. & Cicciù, M. (2019). Molecular Biomarkers Related to Oral Carcinoma: Clinical Trial Outcome Evaluation in a

Literature Review. *Disease markers, 8040361.* https://doi.org/10.1155/2019/8040361.

[21] Kulasingam, V. & Diamandis, E. P. (2008). Strategies for discovering novel cancer biomarkers through utilization of emerging technologies. *Nature clinical practice. Oncology*, *5*(10), 588–599. https://doi.org/10.1038/ncponc1187.

[22] Diamandis, E. P. (2010). Cancer biomarkers: can we turn recent failures into success?. *Journal of the National Cancer Institute, 102*(19), 1462–1467. https://doi.org/10.1093/jnci/djq306.

[23] Nagata, M., Kurita, H., Uematsu, K., Ogawa, S., Takahashi, K., Hoshina, H. & Takagi, R. (2015). Diagnostic value of cyclin-dependent kinase/cyclin-dependent kinase inhibitor expression ratios as biomarkers of locoregional and hematogenous dissemination risks in oral squamous cell carcinoma. *Molecular and clinical oncology, 3*(5), 1007–1013. https://doi.org/10.3892/mco.2015.578.

[24] Lee, D. H. (2018). Practical issues of biomarker-assisted targeted therapy in precision medicine and immuno-oncology era. *ESMO open, 3*(Suppl 1), e000370. https://doi.org/10.1136/esmoopen-2018-000370.

[25] Sethi, S., Ali, S., Philip, P. A. & Sarkar, F. H. (2013). Clinical advances in molecular biomarkers for cancer diagnosis and therapy. *International journal of molecular sciences*, *14*(7), 14771–14784. https://doi.org/10.3390/ijms140714771.

[26] Bhatt, A. N., Mathur, R., Farooque, A., Verma, A. & Dwarakanath, B. S. (2010). Cancer biomarkers - current perspectives. *The Indian journal of medical research*, *132*, 129–149.

[27] Kulasingam, V. & Diamandis, E. P. (2008). Strategies for discovering novel cancer biomarkers through utilization of emerging technologies. *Nature clinical practice. Oncology*, *5*(10), 588–599. https://doi.org/10.1038/ncponc1187.

[28] Ghallab, N. A. & Shaker, O. G. (2017). Serum and salivary levels of chemerin and MMP-9 in oral squamous cell carcinoma and oral premalignant lesions. *Clinical oral investigations*, *21*(3), 937–947. https://doi.org/10.1007/s00784-016-1846-8.

[29] Jiang, T., Xie, P. & Liu, H. (2016). Circulating Anti-Matrix Metalloproteinase-7 Antibodies May Be a Potential Biomarker for Oral Squamous Cell Carcinoma. *Journal of oral and maxillofacial surgery : official journal of the American Association of Oral and Maxillofacial Surgeons*, *74*(3), 650–657. https://doi.org/10.1016/j.joms.2015.09.016.

[30] Xu, H., Yang, Y., Zhao, H., Yang, X., Luo, Y., Ren, Y.,Liu, W. & Li, N. (2016). Serum miR-483-5p: a novel diagnostic and prognostic biomarker for patients with oral squamous cell carcinoma. *Tumor Biology.*, *1*, 447-53.

[31] Malhotra, R., Urs, A. B., Chakravarti, A., Kumar, S., Gupta, V. K. & Mahajan, B. (2016). Correlation of Cyfra 21-1 levels in saliva and serum with CK19 mRNA expression in oral squamous cell carcinoma. *Tumour biology: the journal of the International Society for Oncodevelopmental Biology and Medicine*, *37*(7), 9263–9271. https://doi.org/10.1007/s13277-016-4809-4.

[32] Moergel, M., Kämmerer, P. W., Schnurr, K., Klein, M. O. & Al-Nawas, B. (2012). Spin electron paramagnetic resonance of albumin for diagnosis of oral squamous cell carcinoma (OSCC). *Clinical oral investigations*, *16*(6), 1529–1533. https://doi.org/10.1007/s00784-011-0655-3.

[33] Maclellan, S. A., Lawson, J., Baik, J., Guillaud, M., Poh, C. F. & Garnis, C. (2012). Differential expression of miRNAs in the serum of patients with high-risk oral lesions. *Cancer medicine*, *1*(2), 268–274. https://doi.org/10.1002/cam4.17.

[34] Chen, Y., Azman, S. N., Kerishnan, J. P., Zain, R. B., Chen, Y. N., Wong, Y. L. & Gopinath, S. C. (2014). Identification of host-immune response protein candidates in the sera of human oral squamous cell carcinoma patients. *PloS one*, *9*(10), e109012. https://doi.org/10.1371/journal.pone.0109012.

[35] Tamaki, S., Sanefuzi, N., Kawakami, M., Aoki, K., Imai, Y., Yamanaka, Y., Yamamoto, K., Ishitani, A., Hatake, K. & Kirita, T. (2008). Association between soluble MICA levels and disease stage IV oral squamous cell carcinoma in Japanese patients. *Human*

immunology, *69*(2), 88–93. https://doi.org/10.1016/ j.humimm.2008.01.010.

[36] Tiziani, S., Lopes, V. & Günther, U. L. (2009). Early stage diagnosis of oral cancer using 1H NMR-based metabolomics. *Neoplasia (New York, N.Y.)*, *11*(3), 269. https://doi.org/10.1593/neo.81396.

[37] Gupta, A., Gupta, S. & Mahdi, A. A. (2015). ^{1}H NMR-derived serum metabolomics of leukoplakia and squamous cell carcinoma. *Clinica chimica acta; international journal of clinical chemistry*, *441*, 47–55. https://doi.org/10.1016/j.cca.2014.12.003.

[38] Li, Y., Elashoff, D., Oh, M., Sinha, U., St John, M. A., Zhou, X., Abemayor, E. & Wong, D. T. (2006). Serum circulating human mRNA profiling and its utility for oral cancer detection. *Journal of clinical oncology: official journal of the American Society of Clinical Oncology*, *24*(11), 1754–1760. https://doi.org/10.1200/ JCO.2005.03.7598.

[39] Yu, C. J., Chang, K. P., Chang, Y. J., Hsu, C. W., Liang, Y., Yu, J. S., Chi, L. M., Chang, Y. S. & Wu, C. C. (2011). Identification of guanylate-binding protein 1 as a potential oral cancer marker involved in cell invasion using omics-based analysis. *Journal of proteome research*, *10*(8), 3778–3788. https://doi.org/10.1021/pr2004133.

[40] Shpitzer, T., Hamzany, Y., Bahar, G., Feinmesser, R., Savulescu, D., Borovoi, I., Gavish, M. & Nagler, R. M. (2009). Salivary analysis of oral cancer biomarkers. *British journal of cancer*, *101*(7), 1194–1198. https://doi.org/10.1038/sj.bjc.6605290.

[41] Lallemant, B., Evrard, A., Combescure, C., Chapuis, H., Chambon, G., Raynal, C., Reynaud, C., Sabra, O., Joubert, D., Hollande, F., Lallemant, J. G., Lumbroso, S. & Brouillet, J. P. (2009). Clinical relevance of nine transcriptional molecular markers for the diagnosis of head and neck squamous cell carcinoma in tissue and saliva rinse. *BMC cancer*, *9*, 370. https://doi.org/10.1186/1471-2407-9-370.

[42] Yu, J. S., Chen, Y. T., Chiang, W. F., Hsiao, Y. C., Chu, L. J., See, L. C., Wu, C. S., Tu, H. T., Chen, H. W., Chen, C. C., Liao, W. C., Chang, Y. T., Wu, C. C., Lin, C. Y., Liu, S. Y., Chiou, S. T., Chia, S. L., Chang, K. P., Chien, C. Y., Chang, S. W. & Hartwell, L. H. (2016).

Saliva protein biomarkers to detect oral squamous cell carcinoma in a high-risk population in Taiwan. *Proceedings of the National Academy of Sciences of the United States of America*, *113*(41), 11549–11554. https://doi.org/10.1073/ pnas.1612368113.

[43] Chen, Y. T., Chen, H. W., Wu, C. F., Chu, L. J., Chiang, W. F., Wu, C. C., Yu, J. S., Tsai, C. H., Liang, K. H., Chang, Y. S., Wu, M. & Ou Yang, W. T. (2017). Development of a Multiplexed Liquid Chromatography Multiple-Reaction-Monitoring Mass Spectrometry (LC-MRM/MS) Method for Evaluation of Salivary Proteins as Oral Cancer Biomarkers. *Molecular & cellular proteomics: MCP*, *16*(5), 799–811. https://doi.org/10.1074/mcp.M116.064758.

[44] Hu, S., Arellano, M., Boontheung, P., Wang, J., Zhou, H., Jiang, J., Elashoff, D., Wei, R., Loo, J. A. & Wong, D. T. (2008). Salivary proteomics for oral cancer biomarker discovery. *Clinical cancer research: an official journal of the American Association for Cancer Research*, *14*(19), 6246–6252. https://doi.org/10.1158/1078-0432.CCR-07-5037.

[45] Franzmann, E. J., Reategui, E. P., Carraway, K. L., Hamilton, K. L., Weed, D. T. & Goodwin, W. J. (2005). Salivary soluble CD44: a potential molecular marker for head and neck cancer. *Cancer epidemiology, biomarkers & prevention: a publication of the American Association for Cancer Research, cosponsored by the American Society of Preventive Oncology*, *14*(3), 735–739. https://doi.org/10.1158/1055-9965.EPI-04-0546.

[46] Li, Y., St John, M. A., Zhou, X., Kim, Y., Sinha, U., Jordan, R. C., Eisele, D., Abemayor, E., Elashoff, D., Park, N. H. & Wong, D. T. (2004). Salivary transcriptome diagnostics for oral cancer detection. *Clinical cancer research: an official journal of the American Association for Cancer Research*, *10*(24), 8442–8450. https://doi.org/10.1158/1078-0432.CCR-04-1167.

[47] Pereira, L. H., Reis, I. M., Reategui, E. P., Gordon, C., Saint-Victor, S., Duncan, R., Gomez, C., Bayers, S., Fisher, P., Perez, A., Goodwin, W. J., Hu, J. J. & Franzmann, E. J. (2016). Risk Stratification System for Oral Cancer Screening. *Cancer prevention research (Philadelphia,*

Pa.), *9*(6), 445–455. https://doi.org/10.1158/1940-6207.CAPR-15-0200.

[48] Brinkmann, O., Kastratovic, D. A., Dimitrijevic, M. V., Konstantinovic, V. S., Jelovac, D. B., Antic, J., Nesic, V. S., Markovic, S. Z., Martinovic, Z. R., Akin, D., Spielmann, N., Zhou, H. & Wong, D. T. (2011). Oral squamous cell carcinoma detection by salivary biomarkers in a Serbian population. *Oral oncology*, *47*(1), 51–55. https://doi.org/10.1016/j.oraloncology.2010.10.009.

[49] Elashoff, D., Zhou, H., Reiss, J., Wang, J., Xiao, H., Henson, B., Hu, S., Arellano, M., Sinha, U., Le, A., Messadi, D., Wang, M., Nabili, V., Lingen, M., Morris, D., Randolph, T., Feng, Z., Akin, D., Kastratovic, D. A., Chia, D. & Wong, D. T. (2012). Prevalidation of salivary biomarkers for oral cancer detection. *Cancer epidemiology, biomarkers & prevention: a publication of the American Association for Cancer Research, cosponsored by the American Society of Preventive Oncology*, *21*(4), 664–672. https://doi.org/10.1158/1055-9965.EPI-11-1093.

[50] Rajkumar, K., Nandhini, G., Ramya, R., Rajashree, P., Kumar, A. R. & Anandan, S. N. (2014). Validation of the diagnostic utility of salivary interleukin 8 in the differentiation of potentially malignant oral lesions and oral squamous cell carcinoma in a region with high endemicity. *Oral surgery, oral medicine, oral pathology and oral radiology*, *118*(3), 309–319. https://doi.org/10.1016/ j.oooo.2014.04.008.

[51] Peisker, A., Raschke, G. F., Fahmy, M. D., Guentsch, A., Roshanghias, K., Hennings, J. & Schultze-Mosgau, S. (2017). Salivary MMP-9 in the detection of oral squamous cell carcinoma. *Medicina oral, patologia oral y cirugia bucal*, *22*(3), e270–e275. https://doi.org/10.4317/medoral.21626.

[52] Wang, Q., Gao, P., Cheng, F., Wang, X. & Duan, Y. (2014). Measurement of salivary metabolite biomarkers for early monitoring of oral cancer with ultra performance liquid chromatography-mass spectrometry. *Talanta*, *119*, 299–305. https://doi.org/10.1016/ j.talanta.2013.11.008.

[53] Wei, J., Xie, G., Zhou, Z., Shi, P., Qiu, Y., Zheng, X., Chen, T., Su, M., Zhao, A. & Jia, W. (2011). Salivary metabolite signatures of oral cancer and leukoplakia. *International journal of cancer*, *129*(9), 2207–2217. https://doi.org/10.1002/ijc.25881.

[54] Yuvaraj, M., Aruna, P., Koteeswaran, D., Tamilkumar, P. & Ganesan, S. (2015). Rapid fluorescence spectroscopic characterization of salivary DNA of normal subjects and OSCC patients using ethidium bromide. *Journal of fluorescence*, *25*(1), 79–85. https://doi.org/10.1007/s10895-014-1482-0.

[55] Chuang, A. Y., Chuang, T. C., Chang, S., Zhou, S., Begum, S., Westra, W. H., Ha, P. K., Koch, W. M. & Califano, J. A. (2008). Presence of HPV DNA in convalescent salivary rinses is an adverse prognostic marker in head and neck squamous cell carcinoma. *Oral oncology*, *44*(10), 915–919. https://doi.org/10.1016/j.oraloncology.2008.01.001.

[56] Alison, M. R., Lim, S. M. & Nicholson, L. J. (2011). Cancer stem cells: problems for therapy?. *The Journal of pathology*, *223*(2), 147–161. https://doi.org/10.1002/path.2793.

[57] Bach, P. B., Jett, J. R., Pastorino, U., Tockman, M. S., Swensen, S. J. & Begg, C. B. (2007). Computed tomography screening and lung cancer outcomes. *JAMA*, *297*(9), 953–961. https://doi.org/10.1001/jama.297.9.953.

INDEX

A

B

E

F

G

H

I

L

M

N

O

P

R

S

T

V

W